This report contains the collective views of an international group of experts and does not necessarily represent the decisions or the stated policy of the United Nations Environment Programme, the International Labour Organisation, or the World Health Organization.

**Environmental Health Criteria 149**

# CARBENDAZIM



First draft prepared by IPCS staff, using texts
made available by Dr L.W. Hershberger
and Dr G.T. Arce, Wilmington, Delaware, USA

Published under the joint sponsorship of
the United Nations Environment Programme,
the International Labour Organisation,
and the World Health Organization

World Health Organization
Geneva, 1993

The **International Programme on Chemical Safety (IPCS)** is a joint venture of the United Nations Environment Programme, the International Labour Organisation, and the World Health Organization. The main objective of the IPCS is to carry out and disseminate evaluations of the effects of chemicals on human health and the quality of the environment. Supporting activities include the development of epidemiological, experimental laboratory, and risk-assessment methods that could produce internationally comparable results, and the development of manpower in the field of toxicology. Other activities carried out by the IPCS include the development of know-how for coping with chemical accidents, coordination of laboratory testing and epidemiological studies, and promotion of research on the mechanisms of the biological action of chemicals.

WHO Library Cataloguing in Publication Data

Carbendazim.

(Environmental health criteria ; 149)

1.Benzimidazoles - adverse effects 2.Benzimidazoles - toxicity 3.Fungicides, Industrial - adverse effects 4.Fungicides, Industrial - toxicity I.Series

ISBN 92 4 157149 7 (NLM Classification: WA 240)
ISSN 0250-8634



PRINTED IN FINLAND
93/9738 — VAMMALA — 5500

## CONTENTS

**WHO TASK GROUP ON ENVIRONMENTAL HEALTH CRITERIA FOR BENOMYL AND CARBENDAZIM**

*Members*

Dr G. Burin, Office of Pesticide Programmes, US Environmental Protection Agency, Washington, D.C., USA

Dr R. Cooper, Reproductive Toxicology Branch, US Environmental Protection Agency, Research Triangle Park, North Carolina, USA

Dr I. Desi, Department of Public Health, Albert Szent-Györgyi University Medical School, Szeged, Hungary

Dr S. Dobson, Institute of Terrestrial Ecology, Monks Wood, Abbots Ripton, Huntingdon, United Kingdom

Dr A. Helweg, Department for Pesticide Analysis and Ecotoxicology, Danish Research Service for Plant and Soil Science, Flakkebjerg, Slagelse, Denmark

Dr M. Lotti, Institute of Occupational Medicine, University of Padua, Padua, Italy (*Chairman*)

Dr K. Maita, Toxicology Division, Institute of Environmental Toxicology, Kodaira-Shi, Tokyo, Japan

Dr F. Matsumura, Department of Environmental Toxicology, Institute of Toxicology and Environmental Health, University of California, Davis, California, USA

Dr T.K. Pandita, Microbiology and Cell Biology Laboratory, Indian Institute of Science, Bangalore, India[a]

Dr C. Sonich-Mullin, Environmental Criteria and Assessment Office, US Environmental Protection Agency, Cincinnati, Ohio, USA

Dr P.P. Yao, Institute of Occupational Medicine, Chinese Academy of Preventive Medicine, Beijing, China

[a] Invited but unable to attend the meeting

*Secretariat*

Dr B.H. Chen, International Programme on Chemical Safety, World Health Organization, Geneva, Switzerland (*Secretary*)

Dr L.W. Hershberger, Dupont Agricultural Products, Walker's Mill, Barley Mill Plaza, Wilmington, Delaware, USA

Mr P. Howe, Institute of Terrestrial Ecology, Monks Wood, Abbots Ripton, Huntington, United Kingdom

## NOTE TO READERS OF THE CRITERIA MONOGRAPHS

Every effort has been made to present information in the criteria monographs as accurately as possible without unduly delaying their publication. In the interest of all users of the Environmental Health Criteria monographs, readers are kindly requested to communicate any errors that may have occurred to the Director of the International Programme on Chemical Safety, World Health Organization, Geneva, Switzerland, in order that they may be included in corrigenda.

* * *

A detailed data profile and a legal file can be obtained from the International Register of Potentially Toxic Chemicals, Palais des Nations, 1211 Geneva 10, Switzerland (Telephone No. 7988400 or 7985850).

## ENVIRONMENTAL HEALTH CRITERIA FOR CARBENDAZIM

A WHO Task Group on Environmental Health Criteria for Benomyl and Carbendazim, sponsored by the US Environmental Protection Agency, met in Cincinnati, USA, from 14 to 19 September 1992. On behalf of the host agency, Dr T. Harvey opened the meeting and welcomed the participants. Dr B.H. Chen of the International Programme on Chemical Safety (IPCS) welcomed the participants on behalf of the Director, IPCS, and the three IPCS cooperating organizations (UNEP/ILO/WHO). The Task Group reviewed and revised the draft criteria monograph and made an evaluation of the risks for human health and the environment from exposure to carbendazim.

The first draft of this monograph was prepared by the staff of IPCS, using texts made available by Dr L.W. Hershberger and Dr G.T. Arce, Wilmington, Delaware, USA. The second draft was prepared by Dr L.W. Hershberger and Dr B.H. Chen incorporating comments received following the circulation of the first draft to the IPCS Contact Points for Environmental Health Criteria monographs. Dr M. Lotti (Institute of Occupational Medicine, University of Padua, Italy) made a considerable contribution to the preparation of the final text. Dr B.H. Chen and Dr P.G. Jenkins, both members of the IPCS Central Unit, were responsible for the overall scientific content and technical editing, respectively.

The efforts of all who helped in the preparation and finalization of the monograph are gratefully acknowledged.

Financial support for the meeting was provided by the US Environmental Protection Agency, Cincinnati, USA.

## ABBREVIATIONS

| | |
|---|---|
| a.i. | active ingredient |
| BSP | Bromosulfophthalein |
| HPLC | high-performance liquid chromatography |
| $K_{oc}$ | Distribution coefficient between pesticide adsorbed to soil organic carbon and pesticide in solution |
| $K_{om}$ | Distribution coefficient between pesticide adsorbed to soil organic matter and pesticide in solution |
| NOEC | no-observed-effect concentration |
| NOEL | no-observed-effect level |
| 2-AB | 2-aminobenzimidazole |
| 5-HBC | methyl (5-hydroxy-1H-benzimidazol-2-yl)-carbamate |

# 1. SUMMARY AND CONCLUSIONS

## 1.1 Summary

### 1.1.1 *Identity, physical and chemical properties, and analytical methods*

Carbendazim, a white crystalline solid, is a systemic fungicide belonging to the benzimidazole family. It melts at approximately 250 °C and has a vapour pressure of < 1 x $10^{-7}$ Pa (< 1 x $10^{-9}$ mbar) at 20 °C. Carbendazim is essentially insoluble in water (8 mg/litre solubility) at pH 7 and 20 °C. It is stable under normal storage conditions.

Residual and environmental analyses are performed by extraction with an organic solvent and the extract is purified by a liquid-liquid partitioning procedure. Measurement of residues may be determined by HPLC or immunoassay.

### 1.1.2 *Sources of human and environmental exposure*

Carbendazim is the most widely used member of the benzimidazole family of fungicides. It is formulated as an aqueous dispersion, aqueous suspension, flowable water-dispersible granule and a wettable powder.

### 1.1.3 *Environmental transport, distribution and transformation*

Benomyl is rapidly converted to carbendazim in the environment, with half-lives of 2 and 19 h in water and in soil, respectively. Data from studies on both benomyl and carbendazim are therefore relevant for the evaluation of environmental effects.

Carbendazim is decomposed in the environment with half-lives of 6 to 12 months on bare soil, 3 to 6 months on turf, and half-lives in water of 2 and 25 months under aerobic and anaerobic conditions, respectively. Carbendazim is mainly decomposed by microorganisms; 2-aminobenzimidazole (2-AB) is the major degradation product and is further decomposed by microbial activity. When phenyl-$^{14}$C-labelled benomyl was decomposed, only 9% of the $^{14}$C label was evolved in $CO_2$ during 1 year of incubation, the remaining $^{14}$C being recovered mainly as carbendazim and bound residues. The fate of a possible degradation product (1,2-diaminobenzene) may shed further light on the degradation pathway of benzimidazole fungicides in the environment.

Field and column studies have shown that carbendazim remains in the soil surface layer. No determination of carbendazim adsorption in soil is available, but it is likely to be as strongly adsorbed to soil as benomyl ($K_{oc}$ values ranking from 1000 to 3600). Log $K_{ow}$ values for benomyl and carbendazim are 1.36 and 1.49, respectively.

A risk of leaching was not apparent when this was evaluated in a screening model based on adsorption and persistence data. This statement is supported by analysis of well water in the USA, where carbendazim has not been found in any of 212 wells (limit of detection not available). Surface run-off of benomyl and carbendazim is expected to consist only of fungicide adsorbed to soil particles, and the fungicides are likely to be strongly adsorbed to sediments in the aqueous environment.

Carbendazim is hydrolysed to 2-AB. This is also the primary metabolite in soil and plants.

In animal systems, carbendazim is metabolized to (5-hydroxy-1H-benzimidazol-2-yl)-carbamate (5-HBC) and other polar metabolites, which are rapidly excreted. Carbendazim has not been observed to accumulate in any biological system.

### 1.1.4 Environmental levels and human exposure

There appear to be no environmental monitoring data for carbendazim. However, the following can be summarized from environmental fate studies.

Due to the fact that they are stable for several weeks on plant material, benomyl and carbendazim may become accessible to organisms feeding on leaf litter. Soil and sediments may contain residues of carbendazim for up to 3 years. However, the strong adsorption of carbendazim to soil and sediment particles reduces the exposure for terrestrial and aquatic organisms.

Primary exposure for the general human population will be from residues of benomyl and carbendazim on food crops. Dietary exposure analysis in the USA (combined benomyl and carbendazim) and the Netherlands (carbendazim) estimated the expected mean intake to be about one-tenth of the recommended Acceptable Daily Intake (ADI) of 0.02 mg/kg body weight for benomyl and 0.01 mg/kg body weight for carbendazim.

Occupational exposure during manufacture is below the Threshold Limit Value established for benomyl. Agricultural workers engaged in pesticide mixing and loading or in re-entering benomyl-treated fields are expected to be exposed to dermal contact of a few mg benomyl per h. This type of exposure could be reduced by the use of protective devices. Furthermore, since dermal absorption is expected to be low, the probability of systemic toxicity of benomyl through this route is very low.

### 1.1.5 Kinetics and metabolism

Carbendazim is well absorbed (80-85%) after oral exposure but much less so by dermal exposure. Absorbed carbendazim is metabolized into many compounds within the organism. The main metabolites are 5-HBC and 5,6-HOBC-N-oxides. Minor metabolites are 5,6-DHBC-S and 5,6-DHBC-G.

The tissue distribution of carbendazim showed no bioconcentration. In the rat, the highest concentration after oral carbendazim administration (< 1% of the dose) occurred in the liver. It was distributed as carbendazim in the mitochondria, 5-HBC in the cytostol, and 2-AB in the microsomes. Carbendazim and its metabolites were also found in the kidney of hens and cows; but no significant levels were detected in other tissues. After carbendazim was fed to lactating cows, small amounts of 5-HBC and 4-HBC were found in the milk.

Carbendazim is excreted in the urine and faeces within 72 h after oral dosing in rats.

In rats and mice, high doses of carbendazim, both in the diet and by gavage, affect certain liver microsomal enzymes. Styrene-7,8-hydrolase and epoxide hydrolase were induced whereas 7-hydroxycoumarin O-deethylase activity was found to be reduced. Cytosolic glutathione S-transferase activity was also induced.

### 1.1.6 Effects on laboratory mammals and *in vitro* test systems

#### 1.1.6.1 Single exposure

Carbendazim has low acute toxicity. The $LD_{50}$ values range from > 2000 to 15 000 mg/kg in a wide variety of test animals and routes of administration. However, significant adverse reproductive effects have been noted following a single exposure (see section 1.1.6.5).

### 1.1.6.2 Short-term exposure

Dietary administration of carbendazim for up to 90 days produced slight effects on liver weight in female rats exposed to 360 mg/kg body weight per day. In a 90-day gavage study in the rat, the NOEL was 16 mg/kg per day based on hepatotoxicity. Short-term feeding studies on dogs were not adequate for establishing a NOEL. A 10-day dermal study in the rabbit revealed no systemic toxicity at the only dose tested (200 mg/kg).

### 1.1.6.3 Skin and eye irritation and sensitization

Application to the skin of the rabbit and guinea-pig produced no irritation or skin sensitization. Application to the eyes of rabbits produced moderate or mild conjunctival irritation.

### 1.1.6.4 Long-term exposure

Male and female rats fed 2500 mg/kg diet showed reduced erythrocyte count and haemoglobin and haematocrit values. No liver-related toxicity was noted. Male rats fed 2500 mg/kg diet or more presented a marginal increase in diffuse testicular atrophy and prostatitis. The NOEL in the rat is 500 mg/kg diet. Elevated serum cholesterol and alkaline phosphatase activity and other indications of hepatotoxicity were observed in dogs fed a diet containing 500 mg carbendazim/kg for 1 year or longer. The NOEL in the dog is 300 mg/kg diet.

Male and female mice fed 5000 mg/kg diet showed increased absolute liver weight. There was also significant centrilobular hypertrophy, necrosis and swelling of the liver in male mice fed 1500 mg/kg diet.

### 1.1.6.5 Reproduction, embryotoxicity and teratogenicity

Carbendazim was without adverse effects on reproduction when it was fed to rats in a three-generation reproduction study at levels up to and including 500 mg/kg diet. Male fertility was depressed in rats when carbendazim (200 mg/kg per day) was administered by gavage for 85 days. A dose of 50 mg/kg body weight per day in this study caused a significant decrease in epididymal sperm count.

Following a single oral dose to rats, histological examination revealed early (0-2 days) disruption of spermatogenesis with occlusion of efferent ducts and increased testicular weights at 100 mg/kg body weight. No effect was observed at 50 mg/kg in this single dose study. These effects persisted until day 70 in rats treated with 400 mg/kg.

Carbendazim caused an increase in malformations and anomalies in rats when administered at daily dose levels greater than 10 mg/kg on days 7-16 of gestation. There was a slightly decreased rate of implantation in rabbits administered 20 and 125 mg/kg per day on days 7-19 of gestation and an increased incidence of resorption at 125 mg/kg per day. Maternal toxicity was observed at 20 mg/kg per day and 125 mg/kg per day in the rat and rabbit, respectively.

In addition to decreased pregnancy rate and increased early resorptions in the rat, there were significant reductions in fetal weights at 20 and 90 mg/kg per day and a significant increase in fetal malformations at 90 mg/kg per day. These consisted primarily of hydrocephaly, microphthalmia, anophthalmia, malformed scapulea and axial skeletal malformations (vertebral, rib and sternebral fusions, exencephaly, hemivertebrae and rib hyperplasia). However, in the rabbit there were no significant malformations.

### 1.6.6 *Mutagenicity and related end-points*

Assays in mammalian and non-mammalian systems *in vitro* and *in vivo* and in somatic cells as well as in germ cells show that carbendazim does not interact with DNA, induce point mutation or cause germ cell mutation.

Carbendazim does, however, cause numerical chromosome aberrations (aneuploidy and/or polyploidy) in experimental systems, both *in vitro* and *in vivo*.

### 1.6.7 *Carcinogenicity*

Benomyl and carbendazim feeding resulted in an increase in the incidence of hepatocellular tumours in CD-1 and SPF Swiss mice.

A carcinogenicity study of carbendazim using CD-1 mice showed a statistically significant dose-related increase in the incidence of hepatocellular neoplasia in females. There was also a statistically significant increase in the mid-dose (1500 mg/kg diet) males, but not in the high-dose males because of a high mortality rate. A carcinogenicity study of carbendazim in a genetically related mouse strain, SPF mice (Swiss random strain) at doses of 0, 150, 300 and 1000 mg/kg diet (increased to 5000 mg/kg during the study) showed an increase in the incidence of combined hepatocellular adenomas and carcinomas. A study carried out in NMRKf mice at dose levels of 0, 50, 150, 300 and 1000 mg/kg diet of carbendazim (increased to 5000 mg/kg during the study) showed no carcinogenic effects. Benomyl or carbendazim caused liver tumours in two strains of mice (CD-1 and SPF), both of which have a high spontaneous rate of liver tumours. In contrast, carbendazim is not carcinogenic in NMRKf mice, which have a low spontaneous rate of such tumours.

Carcinogenicity studies of both benomyl and carbendazim in rats were negative.

#### 1.1.6.8 Mechanism of toxicity - mode of action

The biological effects of benomyl and carbendazim result from their interaction with cell microtubules. These structures are involved in vital functions such as cell division, which is inhibited by benomyl and carbendazim. Benomyl and carbendazim toxicities in mammals are linked to microtubular dysfunction.

Benomyl and carbendazim, as well as other benzimidazole compounds, display species-selective toxicity. This selectivity is, at least in part, explained by the different binding of benomyl and carbendazim to tubulins of target and non-target species.

### 1.1.7 Effects on humans

No adverse effects on human health have been reported.

### 1.1.8 Effects on other organisms in the laboratory and field

Carbendazim has little effect on soil microbial activity at recommended application rates. Some adverse effects have been reported for groups of fungi.

The 72-h $EC_{50}$, based on total growth, for the green alga *Selenastrum capricornutum* was calculated to be 1.3 mg/litre; the NOEC was 0.5 mg/litre. The toxicity of carbendazim to aquatic invertebrates and fish varies widely, with 96-h $LC_{50}$ values ranging from 0.007 mg/litre for the channel catfish to 5.5 mg/litre for the bluegill sunfish. In a 21-day test on *Daphnia magna* the onset of reproduction was significantly delayed at 0.025 mg/litre; the NOEC was 0.013 mg/litre.

Carbendazim is toxic to earthworms in laboratory experiments at realistic exposure concentrations and from recommended use in the field. It is "relatively non-toxic" to honey-bees and of low toxicity to birds.

## 1.2 Conclusions

Benomyl causes dermal sensitization in humans. Benomyl and carbendazim represent a very low risk for acute poisoning in humans. Given the current exposures and the low rate of dermal absorption of benomyl and carbendazim, it is unlikely that they would cause systemic toxicity effects either in the general population or in occupationally exposed subjects. These conclusions are drawn from animal data and the limited human data, but these extrapolations are supported by the understanding of the mode of action of carbendazim and benomyl in both target and non-target species.

Further elucidation of the mechanism of toxicity of carbendazim and benomyl in mammals will perhaps enable a better definition of no-observed-effect levels. Binding studies on tubulins of target cells (testis and embryonic tissues) will facilitate inter-species comparisons.

Carbendazim is strongly adsorbed to soil organic matter and persists in soil for up to 3 years. It also persists on leaf surfaces and, therefore, in leaf litter. Earthworms have been shown to be adversely affected (population and reproductive effects) at recommended application rates. There is no information on other soil or litter arthropods that would be similarly exposed.

The high toxicity to aquatic organisms in laboratory tests is unlikely to be seen in the field because of the low bioavailability of sediment-bound residues of carbendazim. However, no information is available on sediment-living species, which would receive the highest exposure.

# 2. IDENTITY, PHYSICAL AND CHEMICAL PROPERTIES, AND ANALYTICAL METHODS

## 2.1 Identity

### 2.1.1 Primary constituent

Common name: Carbendazim (BSI, ISO)

Chemical structure:

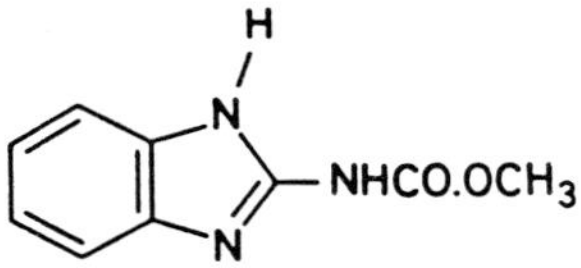

Empirical formula: $C_9H_9N_3O_2$

Relative molecular mass: 191.2

CAS chemical name: Methyl (1H-benzimidazol-2-yl)carbamate

IUPAC chemical name: Methyl benzimidazole-2-ylcarbamate

CAS Registry number: 10605-21-7

Synonyms: carbendazol (ZMAF), methyl-2-benzimidazole carbamate (MBC, MCB, BCM, BMC)

### 2.1.2 Technical product

Major trade names:

Carbendazim, Delsene, Bavistin, Corbel, Konker, Bendazim, Derosal, Kombat, Kemdazin, Carbendor, Hoe 017411, Cekudazim, Equitdazin, Aimcozim (Some of these are formulations with other pesticides.)

| | |
|---|---|
| Purity: | > 98% (FAO specifications) |
| Impurities: | 2,3-diaminophenazine (DAP), 2-amino-3-hydroxyphenazine (HAP) |

## 2.2 Physical and chemical properties

Table 1. Some physical and chemical properties of carbendazim

| | | |
|---|---|---|
| Physical state | Crystalline solid | |
| Colour | White | |
| Odour | Negligible | |
| Melting point/boiling point/flash point | Melts at ~250 °C | |
| Explosion limits | LEL = 0.13 g/litre in air | |
| Vapour pressure | < 1 x $10^{-7}$ Pa (< 1 x $10^{-9}$ mbar) at 20 °C | |
| Density | 0.27 $g/cm^3$ (loose); 0.62 $g/cm^3$ (packed) | |
| Log *n*-octanol/water partition coefficient | 1.49 | |
| Solubility in water (at 20 °C) | pH 4 | 28 mg/litre |
| | pH 7 | 8 mg/litre |
| | pH 8 | 7 mg/litre |
| Solubility in organic solvents | | |
| | Hexane | 0.5 mg/litre |
| | Benzene | 36 mg/litre |
| | Dichloromethane | 68 mg/litre |
| | Ethanol | 300 mg/litre |
| | Dimethylformamide | 5000 mg/litre |
| | Acetone | 300 mg/litre |
| | Chloroform | 100 mg/litre |
| Henry's constant | 1.02 x $10^{-9}$ atm-$m^3$/mol at 20 °C | |

## 2.3 Analytical methods

Methods for determining carbendazim and its by-product residues in plant and animal tissue and in soil involve isolation of the residue by extraction with an organic solvent and purification of the extract by a liquid-liquid partitioning procedure. Measurement of the residues may be determined by procedures using high-speed cation exchange liquid chromatography, reversed phase HPLC, and immunoassay. Recoveries of carbendazim and 2-aminobenzimidazole (2-AB) from various types of soils average 88 and 71%, respectively. The lower limit of sensitivity of the method is 0.05 ppm for each of these components. The recoveries and sensitivities in the case of plant tissues are similar. Table 2 outlines various methods for soil, water, plants and animal tissue.

Table 2. Analytical methods for carbendazim

| Analytical method | Medium | Detection limit | Comments | Reference |
|---|---|---|---|---|
| Strong cation exchange/HPLC | soil | 0.05 mg/kg | acidic methanol extraction converts residual benomyl to carbendazim | Kirkland et al. (1973) |
| Strong cation exchange/HPLC | plant | 0.05 mg/kg | acidic methanol extraction converts residual benomyl to carbendazim | Kirkland et al. (1973) |
| Strong cation exchange/HPLC | animal | 0.01 mg/kg (milk) 0.05 mg/kg (tissue) | acidic aqueous hydrolysis followed by organic extraction converts benomyl to carbendazim and frees metabolites from conjugates | Kirkland (1973) |
| Reversed phase HPLC | water | $9.0 \times 10^{-6}$ g/litre | on-line HPLC with preconcentration; benomyl and carbendazim determined separately | Marvin et al. (1991) |
| Reversed phase HPLC/fluorescence detection | blueberries | 0.03 mg/kg | acidic methanol extraction converts residual benomyl to carbendazim | Bushway et al. (1991) |
| Radioimmunoassay | plant | 0.05-1.0 mg/kg (dependent on crop) | ethyl acetate extraction converts residual benomyl to carbendazim | Newsome & Shields (1981) |
| Enzyme-linked immunosorbent assay (ELISA) | plant | 0.50 mg/kg | ethyl acetate extraction converts residual benomyl to carbendazim | Newsome & Collins (1987) |

# 3. SOURCES OF HUMAN AND ENVIRONMENTAL EXPOSURE

## 3.1 Natural occurrence

Carbendazim does not occur naturally.

## 3.2 Anthropogenic sources

### 3.2.1 Uses

Carbendazim is a fungicide in its own right as well being as the main metabolite of other fungicides such as benomyl and thiophanate-methyl.

Carbendazim is used to control a wide range of fungi, including Ascomycetes, Fungi Imperfecti and numerous Basidiomycetes, which result in plant diseases such as: leaf spots, blotches and blights; fruit spots and rots; sooty molds; scabs; bulb, corn and tuber decays; blossom blights; powdery mildews; certain rusts; and common soilborne crown and root rots. It is used on cereals, cotton, grapes, bananas and other fruit, ornamentals, plantation crops, sugar beet, soybeans, tobacco, turf, vegetables, mushrooms, and many other crops under most climatic conditions worldwide. Registered carbendazim usage specifies rates from 0.2 to 2.0 kg a.i./ha and applications from once per year to spray intervals ranging from 7 to 14 days (FAO/WHO, 1985b; 1988b).

A key limitation to the use of carbendazim and other benzimidazoles is the development of fungal resistance. Resistance management can be achieved by using carbendazim in combination as a tank mix or alternately with other non-benzimidazole fungicides (Delp, 1980; Staub & Sozzi, 1984).

Carbendazim is formulated as an aqueous dispersion, aqueous suspension, flowable water dispersible granules and a wettable powder.

In 1991, the estimated worldwide sales of benomyl was US$ 290 million. This was about 50% of the worldwide market for benzimidazole products. Carbendazim (20%) and thiophanate-methyl (20%) account for most of the rest of the benzimidazole market (County NatWest Woodmac, 1992).

# 4. ENVIRONMENTAL TRANSPORT, DISTRIBUTION AND TRANSFORMATION

## 4.1 Transport and distribution between media

### *4.1.1 Air*

Carbendazim has a vapour pressure of < 1 x $10^{-7}$ Pa (< 1 x $10^{-9}$ mbar) at 20 °C, an aqueous solubility of 8 mg/litre at 20 °C and pH 7, and a Henry's constant of ~1.02 x $10^{-9}$ atm-$m^3$/mol at 20 °C. It is essentially non-volatile from water surfaces.

### *4.1.2 Water*

Anaerobic aquatic degradation studies of [phenyl(U)-$^{14}$C]-benomyl in pond water and sediment showed that more than 98% of the carbendazim residues partitioned into the sediment after 7 days. The half-life of carbendazim was 743 days. After one year 36% of the applied radioactivity was bound to the sediment (Arthur et al., 1989a).

An aerobic aquatic degradation study of [phenyl(U)-$^{14}$C]-benomyl in pond water and sediment showed that carbendazim had a half-life of 61 days under nonsterile conditions. After 30 days, 22% of the applied radioactivity was bound to the sediments and < 1% of the applied radioactivity was evolved as carbon dioxide (Arthur et al., 1989b).

### *4.1.3 Soil*

In greenhouse studies to determine run-off and leaching of [2-$^{14}$C]-carbendazim on soil, a container of Keyport silt loam was treated with labelled carbendazim, at a rate of 11 kg a.i./ha, by spraying the upper one-third (0.093 $m^2$) of the plot and was allowed to stand for 24 h. Artificial rain was then applied (3.75 cm the first day after treatment and 2.5 cm on the third and seventh days). All water that ran off or leached through the soil was collected and analysed for total $^{14}$C. Soil in the plot was divided into layers for analysis, air dried and analysed separately for total $^{14}$C. After each of the three rain applications, 0.05-0.39% of the applied $^{14}$C was found in run-off water; < 0.01% was found in the leach water after the first two artificial rains and 0.19% after the third one. Soil analyses showed that 90.6% of the applied activity remained in the treated area and 93.1% in the top 10 cm of soil (Rhodes & Long, 1983).

### 4.1.4 Leaching

To evaluate the risk of pollution of ground and drainage water, screening models based on adsorption and persistence can be used, together with existing analyses of groundwater samples. Gustafson (1989) proposed the use of the equation GUS = log $T_{½}$ (4 - log $K_{oc}$); GUS values < 1.8 = "improbable leachers", GUS values of 1.8-2.8 = "transition" and GUS values > 2.8 = "probable leachers". For benomyl, $K_{om}$ values of 550, 620, 2100 and 1100 (mean 1093) were found in four different soils (Priester, 1985). A $K_{om}$ of 1093 is equal to a $K_{oc}$ of 1857 since $K_{oc} = K_{om} \times 1.7$. The half-life of 320 days given by Marsh & Arthur (1989) seems in good agreement with field half-lives of 6 to 12 months (Baude et al., 1974).

When the calculation of the GUS value is based on a $K_{oc}$ of 1857 and a $T_{0.5}$ of 320 days, a value of 1.83 is obtained. According to this value, benomyl/carbendazim lies between the "improbable leachers" and "transition", and, therefore, would not be expected to occur in ground water. The adsorption of benomyl and of carbendazim is expected to be of the same order of magnitude since the $K_{ow}$ values are almost identical (log $K_{ow}$ = 1.49 and 1.36 for carbendazim and benomyl, respectively). In groundwater studies in the USA (Parsons & Witt, 1988), benomyl was not found in any of 495 wells tested and carbendazim not in any of 212 wells (detection limit not reported).

In an EEC survey (Fielding, 1992), the presence of carbendazim in groundwater in the Netherlands and in Italy was investigated. Carbendazim was found in one of two samples from the Netherlands (0.1 μg/litre), and the level was above 0.1 μg/litre in 23 of 70 samples in Italy. Detection of the non-polar DDT and lindane in many wells in the Italian study may indicate macropore transport or artifacts such as direct pollution of wells.

### 4.1.5 Crop uptake

Various greenhouse and outdoor tests with carbendazim indicate that it remains on plant surfaces as the major component of the total residue (Baude et al., 1973).

A greenhouse crop-rotation study was undertaken by application of [2-$^{14}$C]carbendazim to a loamy sand soil, followed by aging periods of 30, 120 or 145 days. The crops studied were beets, barley and cabbage. Radioactivity did not accumulate in these crops grown to maturity in a loamy sand soil treated 30 days earlier (1.1 kg a.i./ha) or 120 to 145 days earlier (3.4 kg a.i./ha). Accumulation factors, calculated as the ratio of radioactivity in the crop to that in the corresponding soil, were very low in beet foliage (0.04) and beet roots (0.03), low in cabbage and barley grain (0.2) and ranged from 0.9 to 1.2 in barley straw (Rhodes, 1987).

Alfalfa, soybean and ryegrass, which were grown in 0.028 $m^3$ (1 cu ft) containers in a greenhouse in soil treated with an 80:20 mixture of carbendazim and 2-aminobenzimidazole (2-AB), contained small but detectable residues of both compounds. Both $^{14}C$-labelled and non-labelled mixtures were applied at the rate of 2.2 kg/ha uniformly incorporated in the 0-10 cm layer of soil. In the $^{14}C$ studies, alfalfa contained total $^{14}C$ residues equivalent to 0.13-0.30 mg/kg of carbendazim/2-AB. Soybean plants contained 0.32-0.53 mg/kg and ryegrass (20-183 days after planting) contained 0.09-0.19 mg/kg. Each plant contained approximately equal amounts of carbendazim, 2-AB and a polar unknown fraction. Alfalfa from the non-labelled series contained 0.05 and 0.08 mg/kg, respectively, of carbendazim and 2-AB at the first cutting and < 0.05 mg/kg of each compound at the second and third cuttings. Soybean plants contained < 0.1 mg 2-AB/kg and 0.59 mg carbendazim/kg. Ryegrass from six cuttings (20-149 days after planting) contained 0.08-0.48 mg carbendazim/kg and < 0.05 mg 2-AB/kg. All data were calculated on a fresh weight basis (Rhodes et al., 1983).

## 4.2 Transformation

### 4.2.1 *Soil biodegradation*

Aerobic degradation studies of labelled [2-$^{14}C$]-2-AB, the primary degradation product of carbendazim in soil, showed that $^{14}C$ evolution increased exponentially from 1 to 22 °C, reached a maximum at 22 °C, remained almost constant up to 35 °C, then became almost zero at 40 °C, when the soil water content was 100% of field capacity. At 25 °C, $^{14}C$ evolution increased exponentially with an increase in the field capacity of water from 28 to 94%. These and other results indicate the presence of organisms that are able to decompose 2-AB (Helweg, 1979).

Laboratory studies on two types of soil under anaerobic conditions using [2-$^{14}C$]-carbendazim showed only a small amount of 2-AB (< 0.1%) and no other degradation products (< 0.05%). Re-incorporation of $^{14}C$ into soil humus was indicated by fractionation studies, which showed that the unextracted $^{14}C$ residue was widely distributed in various organic soil components (Han, 1983b).

The persistence of carbendazim was monitored in nonsterile and sterile Keyport silt loam soil after it was treated with [phenyl(U)-$^{14}C$]-benomyl at a concentration of approximately 7.0 mg/kg. Distilled water was added to each sample until it reached 75% of its moisture-holding capacity at 0.33 bar. The soils were incubated in the dark at approximately 25 °C. The nonsterile flasks were sampled after 0.1, 0.2, 1, 3, 7, 14, 30, 60, 120, 270 and 365 days, while samples of sterilized soil were taken after 14, 30, 120, 270 and 365 days. Carbendazim had a half-life of 320 days under nonsterile aerobic conditions (Marsh & Arthur, 1989). This is in close agreement with reported half-lives of 6-12 months for benzimidazoles applied to bare soil (Baude et al., 1974).

After 365 days of incubation, 9% of the $^{14}C$ was evolved as $^{14}CO_2$, 34% could still be recovered as carbendazim, and 36% was not extractable. The total recovery of $^{14}C$ was 88%. In the sterilized soil, the half-life of carbendazim was approximately 1000 days (Marsh & Arthur, 1989).

When the degradation of [2-$^{14}C$]-carbendazim in soil (20 mg/kg) was determined, 33% of added $^{14}C$ was evolved as $^{14}CO_2$ during 270 days. Identical or even faster $^{14}C$ evolution was observed from 2-$^{14}C$-labelled 2-AB (Helweg, 1977). The relatively low $^{14}C$ evolution from phenyl-$^{14}C$-labelled benomyl/carbendazim may be caused by the formation of strongly adsorbed degradation products or compounds that are readily incorporated in soil organic matter. Thus, most of the remaining radioactivity was accounted for in the organic fraction of the soil.

To elucidate the reason for the low $^{14}C$ evolution from phenyl-$^{14}C$-labelled fungicide, the fate of a possible degradation product, 1,2-diaminobenzene, needs to be determined.

In a study on the effect of different factors on the degradation of carbendazim in soil, carbendazim was found to remain in the soil for 120 days. There was 15-29% greater persistence in sterilized soil than nonsterilized ones. *Aspergillus niger tiegh.*, *Penicillum chrysogenum Thom.*, *Mucor* sp and 2 bacteria (*Bacillus* spp.) alone or in combination degraded the fungicide faster. Bacteria were most efficient, and there was faster degradation during the first 20 days. High temperature, acidic pH and higher moisture level in soil in the presence of microbes all let to faster degradation of the fungicide. Soil pre-treatment with microbes resulted in rapid degradation (Gupta & Sharma, 1989).

Soils collected from various fields, which had a history of carbendazim application, showed increased carbendazim degradation rates. Low initial doses of carbendazim sufficed to condition soil with no history of carbendazim application to rapid degradation. Previous application of the fungicide was not the only means of inducing the phenomenon. When soil with a history of carbendazim-treatment was mixed with untreated soil, the ability to accelerate degradation was observed in the entire soil volume. This capacity was maintained in soil for over 2 years without intermediate carbendazim application (Yarden et al., 1987).

Bean plants grown to maturity in Delaware, USA, contained less than 0.1 mg/kg total $^{14}C$ residue in the edible beans following two foliar applications of 1 kg a.i./ha of [2-$^{14}C$]-carbendazim (as Delsene 50% WP) at 25% and 50% bloom. Total $^{14}C$ residues in the bean foliage decreased from about 5 mg/kg one week after the second spraying to 0.2 mg/kg three weeks later. The total $^{14}C$ residue in edible beans was less than 0.1 mg/kg one week after the second spraying. Of the total $^{14}C$ in the edible beans and foliage, 89-95% was intact free carbendazim and 2-8% was free 2-AB. An additional 1-3% of the $^{14}C$ was found as $\beta$-glycosidic conjugates of carbendazim and 2-AB (Han, 1983a).

Chiba & Veres (1981) applied benomyl to apple trees as Benlate 50% WP at a rate of 1.7 kg/ha. Three successive applications were made in 1977 and a single spray was applied in 1979. Between 3 and 7 days after application there was a marked reduction of about 50% in benomyl residues from an initial level of about 110 mg/kg. This fall in benomyl was accompanied by a doubling in the level of carbendazim residues over the same period due to benomyl degradation to carbendazim. Within 46 days of the single application in 1979, benomyl residues fell to 0.63 mg/kg foliage and carbendazim was present at 1.2 mg/kg. Following the three sprayings in 1977 (at 0, 13 and 27 days after the initial application), residue levels were 2.6 and 17.1 mg/kg foliage for benomyl and carbendazim 83 days after the first spraying. Both experiments showed an exponential fall in benomyl residues but the rate of decline was much slower in the case of the more persistent metabolite.

### 4.2.2 *Abiotic degradation*

The hydrolytic stability of carbendazim at pH 5, 7, and 9 and a nominal temperature of 22, 50 and 70 °C was studied at intervals up to 30 days. Elevation of temperature and pH increased carbendazim degradation. The half-life calculated for the degradation of carbendazim at pH 5 and at 22, 50 and 70 °C was 457, 108, and 29 days, respectively. At pH 7 and at 50 and 70 °C the half-life was 43 and 12 days (no appreciable decline at 22 °C). The half-life at pH 9 and at 22, 50, and 70 °C was 22, 1.4 and 0.3 days, respectively (Purser, 1987).

Carbendazim was exposed to sunlight for 30 h (as a residue on silica gel G) and less then 10% was lost after exposure. Photo-oxidation of the benzene ring of carbendazim was the predominant reaction with some guanine, carbomethoxyguanine, and carbomethoxyurea detected. When carbendazim was applied to the leaves of corn plants and exposed to sunlight for 18 h, no photolysis products were detected in the extracts of plants (Fleeker & Lacy, 1977).

### 4.2.3 *Bioaccumulation*

Bluegill sunfish (*Lepomis macrochirus*) were exposed to radiolabelled carbendazim concentrations of 0.018 or 0.17 mg/litre for 4 weeks in a dynamic study designed to measure the bioaccumulation of $^{14}C$ residues in edible tissue, viscera, remaining carcass and whole fish. A two-week depuration phase followed the exposure phase. Results were similar at the two exposure concentrations, the peak whole fish bioconcentration factors (BCFs) being 27 and 23 at the low and high exposure levels, respectively. The radioactivity was concentrated more in the viscera than in other tissues, the peak viscera BCFs being 460 and 380 for the low and high exposure levels, respectively. Very little bioconcentration occurred in the muscle tissue (BCF = < 4) or the remaining carcass (BCF = < 7). During the 14-day depuration phase, > 94% of the peak level of radioactivity was lost from the whole fish, viscera and muscle. The rate of loss from the carcass tissue was lower (77% and 82% loss for the low and high exposure levels, respectively) (Hutton et al., 1984).

When rainbow trout (*Oncorhynchus mykiss*), channel catfish (*Ictalurus punctatus*) and bluegill sunfish (*Lepomis macrochirus*) were injected intraperitoneally with carbendazim, branchial and biliary excretion were the major pathways for the elimination

(Palawski & Knowles, 1986). In a separate experiment, the three fish species were exposed to 45 μg carbendazim/litre for 96 h, except in the case of catfish, which were exposed for 48 h. This was followed by a 96-h depuration phase. Rainbow trout had the highest uptake rate constant (1.78 per h) and bioconcentration factor (159) of the three species. Much less carbendazim was accumulated by channel catfish than by the other two species, but this residue level (0.44 μg/g) appeared to be lethal after 48 h of exposure. The elimination rate constant and the biological half-life of carbendazim were similar for rainbow trout and bluegill sunfish. However, the elimination rate constant was greater and the biological half-life shorter in channel catfish (13 h) than in the other two species.

# 5. ENVIRONMENTAL LEVELS AND HUMAN EXPOSURE

## 5.1 Environmental levels

### *5.1.1 Air, water and soil*

The environmental levels in air, water and soil are discussed in detail in chapter 4.

### *5.1.2 Food and feed*

Levels of carbendazim in food and feed are indicated in section 5.2.

### *5.1.3 Terrestrial and aquatic organisms*

Carbendazim levels in terrestrial and aquatic organisms are discussed in detail in chapters 4 and 6.

## 5.2 General population exposure

The principal exposure of the general population to carbendazim is through dietary exposure. It was recommended by the Joint FAO/WHO Meeting on Pesticide Residues (JMPR) (FAO/WHO, 1985a) that all maximum residue limits (MRLs) for benomyl, thiophanate-methyl and carbendazim be listed as carbendazim (Tables 3 and 4).

### *5.2.1 Sweden*

Monitoring data from Sweden are shown in Table 5 (FAO/WHO, 1988b). No further analysis to determine dietary intake was performed.

### *5.2.2 The Netherlands*

Over a period of two years (June 1976 to July 1978), "market basket" samples for 16- to 18-year-old males, including 126 different food items, were purchased every two months. This age group was chosen by the authors under the assumption that they had the greatest food consumption. The food was prepared for eating (including cooking) and combined in 12 different commodity groups, and the concentrations of 78 different

Table 3. Benomyl/carbendazim/thiophanate-methyl residues in food in Sweden[a]

| Samples | Swedish/imported | No. of samples | Samples with residues ≥0.20 mg/kg | Residue level (mg/kg) | Median value (mg/kg) |
|---|---|---|---|---|---|
| **1986** | | | | | |
| Pineapples | imported | 3 | 1 | 0.69 | |
| Grapes | imported | 20 | 3 | 0.17 0.35 | 0.26 |
| Strawberries | imported | 7 | 1 | 0.29 | |
| Mangoes | imported | 17 | 4 | 0.20-1.82 | 0.70 |
| Papayas | imported | 5 | 2 | 0.25-0.45 | |
| Pears | Swedish | 17 | 3 | 0.32-0.62 | 0.43 |
| | imported | 45 | 7 | 0.20-0.45 | 0.34 |
| Apples | Swedish | 78 | 17 | 0.20-0.72 | 0.40 |
| | imported | 91 | 30 | 0.21-0.74 | 0.39 |
| **1987** | | | | | |
| Grapes | imported | 28 | 3 | 0.52-0.87 | 0.60 |
| Strawberries | imported | 7 | | 0.23 | |
| Mangoes | imported | 14 | 5 | 0.29-1.30 | 0.66 |
| Papayas | imported | 4 | 2 | 0.86-1.14 | |
| Pears | Swedish | 14 | 1 | 0.52 | |
| | imported | 62 | 13 | 0.21-0.45 | 0.29 |
| Apples | Swedish | 61 | 25 | 0.20-1.17 | 0.45 |
| | imported | 94 | 12 | 0.21-0.82 | 0.36 |

[a] From: FAO/WHO (1988b)

Table 4. National Maximum Residue Limits (mg/kg) for certain commodities[a]

| | banana | cereal | cherries | citrus | bean | cucum-ber | peach | pome fruit | straw-berries | grapes |
|---|---|---|---|---|---|---|---|---|---|---|
| Australia | 1 | 0.05 | 5 | 10 | 3 | 3 | 5 | 5 | 6 | 2 |
| Austria | 0.2 | 0.5 | | 7 | 1 | 0.5 | | 2 | 1.5 | 3 |
| Belgium | 2 | 0.5 | 2 | | 2 | 0.5 | 2 | 5 | 5 | 2 |
| Brazil | 1 | 0.5 | 10 | 10 | 2 | 0.5 | 10 | 5 | 5 | 10 |
| Bulgaria | | 0.5 | 10 | | | | | 5 | 5 | 10 |
| Canada | | | 5 | 10 | 1 | 0.5 | 10 | 5 | 5 | 5 |
| Denmark | 2 | 0.1 | 2 | 5 | 2 | 2 | 2 | 2 | 5 | 5 |
| France | 1 | | | 1.5 | | | | 6 | | |
| Finland | 0.2 | | 1 | 2 | 0.5 | 0.5 | 1 | 1 | 1 | |
| Germany | 0.2 | 0.5 | 2 | 7 | 1 | 0.5 | | 2 | 2 | 3 |
| Hungary | | | 2 | | | 1 | | | | |
| Israel | | | 10 | 10 | | | 10 | 5 | | 10 |
| Italy | | 0.5 | | | | | 0.5 | 1 | | 1 |

Table 4 (contd).

| | banana | cereal | cherries | citrus | bean | cucum-ber | peach | pome fruit | straw-berries | grapes |
|---|---|---|---|---|---|---|---|---|---|---|
| Mexico | | | | 10 | 2 | 1 | 15 | 7 | 5 | 10 |
| Netherlands | 3 | 0.1 | 3 | 4 | 3 | 3 | 3 | 3 | 3 | 3 |
| New Zealand | 5 | 1 | 5 | 5 | 2 | 2 | 5 | 5 | 5 | 5 |
| Spain (guidelines) | 1 | 0.5 | 5 | 7 | 2 | 2 | 5 | 5 | 1 | 5 |
| Switzerland | 1 | 0.2 | 3 | 7 | 0.2 | 0.1 | 3 | 3 | 3 | 3 |
| United Kingdom (proposed) | 1 | 0.5 | | 10 | | 0.5 | 10 | 5 | 5 | 10 |
| USA | 1 | 0.2 | 15 | 10 | 2 | 1 | 15 | 7 | 5 | 10 |
| USSR | 1 | 0.5 | 10 | 10 | 2 | 0.5 | 10 | 5 | 5 | 5 |
| Yugoslavia | | 0.1 | | 7 | 0.5 | 0.1 | | 2 | 0.5 | 2 |

[a] From: FAO/WHO (1988a)

Table 5. Proposed Maximum Residue Limits for carbendazim from any source[a]

| Commodity | MRL (mg/kg) | Application[b] |
|---|---|---|
| Apricot | 10[c] | B,C |
| Asparagus | 0.1[d] | B,T |
| Avocado | 0.5 | B |
| Banana | 1[c] | B,C,T |
| Barley straw and fodder, dry | 2 | B |
| Bean fodder | 50 | C |
| Beans, dry | 2 | B |
| Berries and other small fruit | 5 | B,C,T |
| Brussel sprouts | 0.5 | B |
| Broad bean | 2 | T |
| Carrot | 5[c] | C,T |
| Cattle meat | 0.1[d] | B |
| Celery | 2 | B,C |
| Cereal grains | 0.5 | B,C,T |
| Cherries | 10[c] | B,C,T |
| Citrus fruits | 10[c] | B,C,T |
| Coffee beans | 0.1[d] | C |
| Common bean[e] | 2 | C |
| Cucumber | 0.5 | B,C,T |
| Eggs (poultry) | 0.1[d] | B,T |
| Egg plant | 0.5 | C |
| Gherkin | 2 | C,T |
| Hops, dry | 50 | C |
| Lettuce, head | 5 | B,C,T |
| Mango | 2 | B |
| Melons, except watermelons | 2[c] | B,C |
| Milk | 0.1[d] | B |
| Mushrooms | 1 | B,C,T |
| Nectarine | 2 | B |
| Onion, bulb | 2 | C,T |
| Peach | 10[c] | B,C,T |
| Peanut | 0.1[d] | B,C |
| Peanut fodder | 5 | B,C |

Table 5 (contd).

| Commodity | MRL (mg/kg) | Application[b] |
|---|---|---|
| Peppers | 5 | C |
| Pineapple | 20[c] | B |
| Plums (including prunes) | 2[c] | B,C,T |
| Pome fruit | 5[c] | B,C,T |
| Potato | 3[c,f] | B,C |
| Poultry meat | 0.1[d] | B,T |
| Rape seed | 0.05[d] | C |
| Rice straw and fodder, dry | 15 | B,C,T |
| Sheep meat | 0.1[d] | B |
| Soya bean, dry | 0.2 | C |
| Soya bean fodder | 0.1[d] | C |
| Squash, summer | 0.5 | B |
| Sugar beet | 0.1[d] | B,C,T |
| Sugar beet leaves on tops | 10 | B,C,T |
| Swede[g] | 0.1[d] | C |
| Sweet potato | 1 | B |
| Taro | 0.1[d] | B |
| Tomato | 5 | B,C,T |
| Tree nuts | 0.1[d] | B |
| Wheat straw and fodder, dry | 5 | B |
| Winter squash | 0.5 | B |

[a] From: FAO/WHO (1988b)
[b] B = benomyl; C = carbendazim; T = thiophanate-methyl
[c] MRL based on post-harvest use
[d] At or about the limit of detection
[e] JMPR recommended 2 mg/kg for dry, dwarf, lima and snap beans. These are all covered by "VP 0526, Common bean" and "VP 0071, Beans, dry" in the new classification
[f] washed before analysis
[g] Described as rutabagas in 1983 recommendation

chemical pesticides were determined. Using concentrations found in the total diet samples, the daily intakes were calculated. For this sub-population, the maximum intake of carbendazim was 0.6 mg/day (calculated using the detection limit as the concentration of the non-detectable residues) and the average dietary intake was

0.05 mg/day. The recommended ADI is 0-0.01 mg/kg body weight (FAO/WHO, 1985a), corresponding to 0.6 mg/day for a 60-kg adult. Therefore, the maximum intake is at the recommended ADI, whereas the average intake is 12 times below the recommended ADI (de Vos et al., 1984).

### 5.2.3 *National maximum residue limits*

National MRLs for certain commodities are listed in Table 4 (FAO/WHO, 1988a).

A complete list of MRLs for carbendazim, including new proposals and an indication of the source of the data (application of benomyl, carbendazim, or thiophanate-methyl) on which the MRL is based, is given in Table 5 (FAO/WHO, 1988b).

## 5.3 Occupational exposure during manufacture, formulation, or use

### 5.3.1 *Exposure during manufacture*

Levels of carbendazim, monitored as worker inhalation exposure, in a major manufacturing facility (Du Pont) were reviewed from 1986 to 1989. The average level of carbendazim was less than 0.3 mg/m$^3$. Table 6 lists established inhalation exposure limits for benomyl and carbendazim.

### 5.3.2 *Exposure during use*

Although no studies have been performed with carbendazim, potential dermal and respiratory exposure to benomyl wettable powder formulation in actual-use situations was determined for tank loading and mixing for aerial application, re-entry into treated crops, and home use (garden, ornamental and greenhouse). For crop treatments, approximately 17 kg benomyl (formulation) was handled per cycle. Maximum exposure occurred in the loading and mixing operation for aerial application, where dermal exposure was 26 mg benomyl per mixing cycle, primarily to hands and forearms (90%), and respiratory exposure averaged 0.08 mg benomyl. Re-entry data revealed dermal and respiratory exposures of 5.9 mg/h and < 0.002 mg/h, respectively. Home-use situations (application of 7 to 8 litres benomyl in hand-held compressed air sprayers) produced exposures of 1 mg and 0.003 mg per application cycle for the dermal and respiratory routes, respectively (Everhart & Holt 1982).

Table 6. Established inhalation exposure limits[a]

| Country and agency | Compound | TWA[b] (mg/m$^3$) | STEL[c] (mg/m$^3$) |
|---|---|---|---|
| Australia | benomyl | 10 | - |
| Belgium | benomyl | 10 | - |
| Denmark | benomyl | 5 | - |
| Finland | benomyl | 10 | 30 |
| France | benomyl | 10 | - |
| Switzerland | benomyl | 10 | - |
| United Kingdom | benomyl | 10 | 15 |
| USA: ACGIH[d] | benomyl | 10 | - |
| USA: NIOSH[e]/OSHA[f] | benomyl | 10 (inhalable dust) | - |
| USA: NIOSH/CSHA | benomyl | 5 (respirable dust) | - |
| USSR | carbendazim | - | 0.1 |

[a] From: ILO (1991)
[b] Time-weighted average
[c] Short-term exposure limit
[d] American Conference of Governmental Industrial Hygienists
[e] National Institute of Occupational Safety and Health
[f] Occupational Safety and Health Administration

# 6. KINETICS AND METABOLISM

Carbendazim is extensively metabolized by animals as described in detail in section 6.3. Metabolite names and structures are given in Table 7, Fig. 1 and Fig. 2.

## 6.1 Absorption

Male albino rats were orally administered a single $^{14}C$-carbendazim dose of 12 mg/kg as a solution in diethyl glycol-ethanol. Based on urinary excretion of $^{14}C$-carbendazim and its metabolites, 5-HBC and 2-AB, the absorption was determined to be about 85% (Krechniak & Klosowska, 1986).

In a study by Monson (1990), young male and female Sprague-Dawley rats were administered a single dose via gavage with $^{14}C$-radiolabelled [phenyl(U)-$^{14}C$]-carbendazim (94% pure, suspended in corn oil) at either a low (50 mg/kg) or a high (1000 mg/kg) dose, and excretion of the radiolabel was monitored every 12 h for 72 h. Most of the radioactivity was excreted by 72 h. The percentages of originally administered radioactivity (i.e. $^{14}C$-carbendazim equivalent) recovered were: a) in urine, 61.7 (male), 53.8 (female) for low dose, 41.4 (male) and 40.7 (female) for high dose; and b) in faeces, 24.4 (male), 33.2 (female) for low dose and 61.9 (male) and 69.5 (female) for high dose. The author concluded that: a) > 98% of the administered dose was recovered in urine and faeces in all test groups; and b) the absorption efficiency of carbendazim was approximately 80% of the actual administered dose for all dose levels, based on the level of radioactivity appearing in urine and the sum of all metabolites appearing in faeces as the result of hepatic metabolism (Monson, 1990).

## 6.2 Distribution and accumulation

In a rat gavage study, [phenyl(U)-$^{14}C$]-carbendazim was administered to Sprague-Dawley rats (five rats per sex per group) using three dosing regimes: a single oral dose of 50 mg/kg; a single oral dose of 50 mg/kg following pre-conditioning gavage of non-labelled carbendazim (50 mg/kg) for 14 days; and a single oral dose of 1000 mg/kg. All rats were sacrificed 72 h after the last dose. Tissue distribution data showed lack of bioconcentration of radiolabelled compound. The highest concentrations of radio-labelled tissue residues (less than 1% of the dose) were detected in the residual carcass and liver (Monson, 1990). This study is discussed in detail in sections 6.3 and 6.4.

Table 7. Carbendazim and its metabolites in animals[a]

| Code name | Chemical name |
|---|---|
| Carbendazim (MBC) | methyl (1-H-benzimidazol-2-yl)carbamate |
| 5-HBC | methyl (5-hydroxy-1H-benzimidazol-2-yl) carbamate |
| 4-HBC | methyl (4-hydroxy-1H-benzimidazol-2-yl) carbamate |
| 5-HBC-S[b] | 2-[(methoxycarbonyl)amino]-1H-benzimidazol-5-yl hydrogen sulfate |
| 5-HBC-G[c] | [2-[(methoxycarbonyl)amino]-1H-benzimidazol-5-yl] β-D-glucopyranosiduronic acid |
| MBC-4,5-epoxide | |
| MBC-5,6-epoxide | |
| MBC-4,5-dihydrodiol | (4,5-dihydro-4,5-dihydroxy-1H-benzimidazol-2-yl) carbamate |
| MBC-5,6-dihydrodiol | (5,6-dihydro-5,6-dihydroxy-1H-benzimidazol-2-yl) carbamate |
| MBC-4,5-diol | |
| MBC-5,6-diol | |
| 5-OH-6-GS-MBC[d] | S-[5,6-dihydro-5-hydroxy-2-(methoxycarbonyl amino)-1H-benzimidazol-4-yl]glutathione |
| 5-OH-4-GS-MBC | S-[4,5-dihydro-5-hydroxy-2-(methoxycarbonyl amino)-1H-benzimidazol-4-yl]glutathione |
| 5,6-HOBC-N-oxide | methyl (6-hydroxy-5-oxo-5H-benzimidazol-2-yl)-carbamate-N-oxide |
| 5,6-HOBC-N-oxide-G | [2-[(methoxycarbonyl)amino]-6-oxo-6H-benzimidazol-5-yl] β-D-glucopyranosiduronic acid-N-oxide |
| 5,6-DHBC | methyl (5,6-dihydroxy-1H-benzimidazol-2-yl) carbamate |
| 5,6-DHBC-G | [6-hydroxy-2-[(methoxycarbonyl)amino]-1H-benzimidazol-5-yl] β-D-glucopyranosiduronic acid |

Table 7 (contd).

| Code name | Chemical name |
|---|---|
| 5,6-DHBC-S | 6-hydroxy-2-[(methoxycarbonyl)amino]-1H-benzimidazol-5-yl 5-(hydrogen sulfate) |
| 2-AB | 2-aminobenzimidazole |
| 2-AB dihydrodiol | 2-amino-4,5-dihydro-4,5-dihydroxy-1H-benzimidazol |
| 5-HAB | 5-hydroxy-2-aminobenzimidazole |

[a] From: Krechniak & Klosowska (1986); Monson (1986, 1990)
[b] S = conjugate with sulfuric acid
[c] G = conjugate with glucuronic acid
[d] GS = conjugate with glutathione

In a study by Krechniak & Klosowska (1986), male albino rats were administered by gavage a single dose of 12 mg carbendazim per kg and the distribution of carbendazim and its metabolites among subcellular liver fractions was determined 1.5 h after dosing. The distribution was not uniform and was not dependent on the lipid content of the fractions. The highest relative concentration of unchanged carbendazim was in the mitochondria. The highest relative concentration of 5-HBC was in the cytosol and that of 2-AB was in the microsomes.

Ten hens were individually dosed for six consecutive days with 0.625 mg [2-$^{14}$C]-carbendazim at a rate equivalent to 5 mg/kg in the average total daily feed. An additional 10 hens were dosed daily with 12.5 mg at a rate equivalent to 120 mg/kg in the average total daily feed. The hens were sacrificed 24 h after the sixth dose and muscle, kidney, liver and fat were sampled. Carbendazim was extensively metabolized to 5-HBC and methyl (4,5-dihydro-4,5-dihydroxy-1H-benzimidazol-2-yl) carbamate. The concentration of radioactivity, calculated as mg carbendazim per kg, in the high-dose hens was 2.63 (liver), 1.74 (kidney), 0.06 (thigh muscle), 0.05 (breast muscle), 0.03 (fat) and 0.63 (day-6 eggs). Approximately 73% of the total radioactivity in the day-6 eggs was identified as 5-HBC (0.26 mg/kg) and unchanged carbendazim (0.15 mg/kg) (Monson, 1986).

In another feeding study, groups of 20 hens were fed carbendazim daily at levels of 0, 5, 15 and 100 mg/kg diet for 28 days. Eggs were collected daily and faeces once a week. After 28 days, 15 hens in each group were sacrificed and samples taken for analysis. The remaining hens were fed a carbendazim-free diet for a further week and then sacrificed. The majority of the material fed was rapidly eliminated as parent compound or as 5-HBC. The only residues found in any of the samples of blood, fat, liver, kidney, tissue or eggs were in the eggs from the 100-mg/kg group. However, the residues (up to 0.1 mg carbendazim/kg and 0.36 mg 5-HBC/kg each) decreased to < 0.05 mg/kg within 4 days of withdrawal of treatment (Eckert et al., 1985).

A lactating Holstein cow was dosed by capsule twice daily (483 mg [2-$^{14}$C]-carbendazim each dose), equivalent to 50 mg/kg in the average total daily feed, for five consecutive days. Samples of milk were collected at each dosing. Approximately 17 h after the tenth dose, the cow was sacrificed. Small amounts of radioactivity corresponding to carbendazim or its metabolites were found in the liver (2.62 mg/kg) and kidney (0.45 mg/kg), but no significant amounts (< 0.09 mg/kg) were detected in other tissues or fat. Only 2.7% of the liver radioactivity was 5-HBC whereas 41% and 3% of the kidney radioactivity corresponded to 5-HBC and 4-HBC, respectively. $^{14}$C residue levels in the milk averaged 0.25 mg/kg (calculated as carbendazim) of which 0.11 mg/kg was 5-HBC and 0.05 mg/kg 4-HBC. No carbendazim (< 0.01 mg/kg) was detected in the milk (Monson, 1985).

Twelve non-lactating female goats were administered a feed-rate-equivalent [phenyl(U)-$^{14}$C]-carbendazim dose of at least 50 mg/kg (range: 50-101 mg/kg) once a day for up to 30 days. A plateau of $^{14}$C residues in the liver was achieved within 2 weeks of dose initiation and was calculated to be 9.48 mg/kg of liver (group mean of the total radiolabelled liver residues for goats sacrificed 2, 3 and 4 weeks after initiation of dosing). The total $^{14}$C residue levels in the liver decreased to 5.17, 3.55 and 1.67 mg/kg at 1, 2 and 3 weeks, respectively, after discontinuing dosing. Based on this data, the elimination half-life for the total $^{14}$C residues from the liver was calculated to be approximately 9 days. The half-life for removal of carbendazim from the general circulation, based on $^{14}$C-carbendazim equivalent whole blood levels, was approximately 10 h. The results of this study suggest that levels of carbendazim-derived residues do not continue to accumulate beyond 2 weeks when goats are exposed to a constant feed-level of 50 mg carbendazim/kg. Furthermore, discontinuation of exposure results in a clearing of residues from the liver (Johnson, 1988).

## 6.3 Metabolic transformation

In a rat gavage study, carbendazim was found to be extensively metabolized. Three dosing regimes (five rats of each sex per group) were used: a single oral dose of 50 mg/kg (low dose); a single oral dose of 50 mg/kg following pre-conditioning gavage with non-radiolabelled carbendazim of 50 mg/kg for 14 days (pre-conditioned low dose); and a single oral dose of 1000 mg/kg (high dose). The 48-h urine from the low-dose and the high-dose rats, and the 14-day urine from the pre-conditioned low-dose group were collected. The total recovery from urine was 61.5 and 61.7% of given doses for the low-dose and pre-conditioned low-dose male groups, 53.2 and 59.3% for the low-dose and pre-conditioned low-dose female groups, and 39 and 41% for both male and female high-dose groups, respectively. 5-HBC-S (21-43% of given dose) was identified as the main metabolite, except in the case of the pre-conditioned low-dose and the high-dose female rat groups (5.5-10%), while in all female rat groups 5,6-HOBC-N-oxide-G (10-19%) was predominant. Both 5,6-DHBC-S and 5,6-DHBC-G were identified as minor metabolites.

In the same study, the faeces were collected at the same periods as the urine. The total recovery from faeces was about 24% for the low-dose and pre-conditioned low-dose male groups, 33-38% for the low-dose and pre-conditioned low-dose female groups, and higher (> 60%) for both male and female high-dose groups. Unchanged carbendazim was about 10-15% of the given dose in the faeces of high-dose rats (Monson, 1990). The proposed metabolic pathway for carbendazim in rats is given in Fig. 1.

NMRI mice and Wistar rats of both sexes were given carbendazim, via gavage, as a single dose of 3 and 300 mg/kg, respectively. Urine was collected during the first 6 h, after which the animals were killed. Almost all the metabolites in urine were conjugated with sulfuric acid. Cleavage of these conjugates by $\beta$-glucuronidase/arylsulfatase released 5-HBC as the only metabolite extractable from water. Mouse urine contained a greater amount of compounds that remained polar after enzyme treatment than the corresponding urine of rats. Analyses revealed no sex differences (Dorn et al., 1983).

In a further study, male albino rats were administered a single intravenous dose of 12 mg carbendazim/kg as a solution in diethylene-glycol. The composition of the measured radioactivity in urine 12 h after dosing was 94% as 5-HBC, 3% as 2-AB, and 3% as carbendazim (Krechniak & Klosowska, 1986).

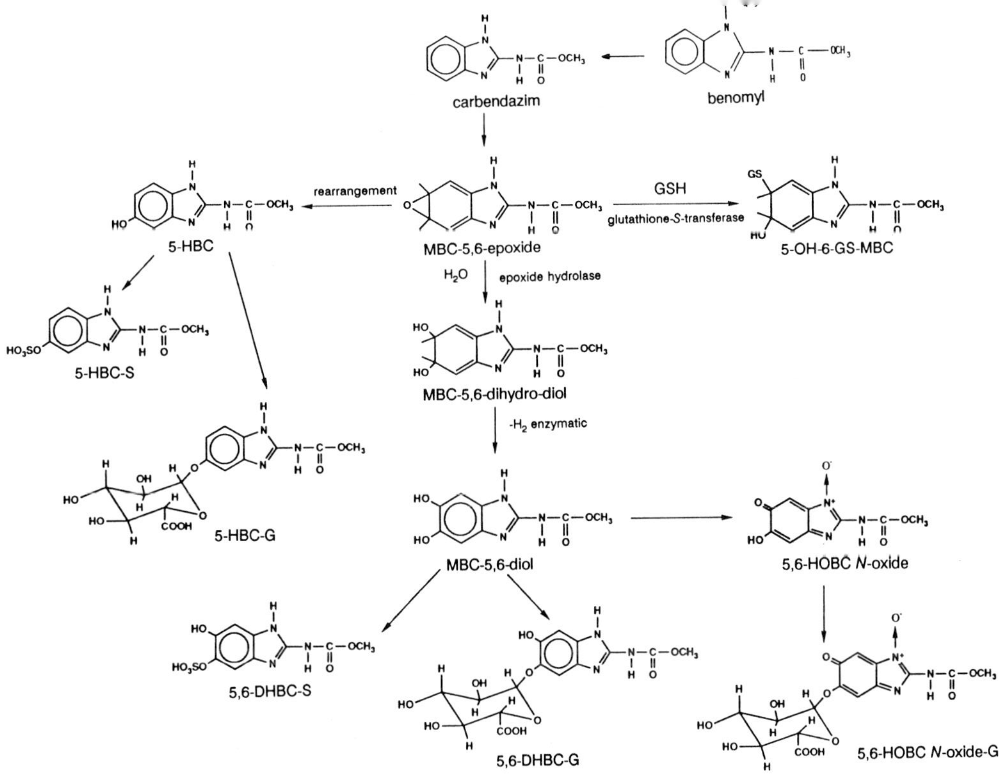


Fig. 1. Proposed metabolic pathway for carbendazim in rats (From: Monson, 1990)

In hens dosed with [2-$^{14}$C]-carbendazim (5 and 120 mg/kg in the daily feed), carbendazim was metabolized to 5-HBC, 4-HBC, 4,5-dihydrodiol-MBC and its sulfuric acid conjugate, and also to 2-AB (Monson, 1986). The proposed metabolic pathway in laying hens is given in Fig. 2.

The metabolic fate of carbendazim in the liver was examined in non-lactating female goats administered a feed-rate-equivalent [phenyl(U)-$^{14}$C]-carbendazim dose of 50 mg/kg once a day for 30 days. Extraction of liver homogenate from goats sacrificed 4 weeks after initiation of dosing, i.e. when the $^{14}$C residues in the liver had reached a plateau, indicated that the major ethyl-acetate-extractable and identifiable radiolabelled residues in the liver were 5-HBC (2 to 3 mg/kg) and carbendazim (approximately 0.2 mg/kg). Bound non-extractable $^{14}$C residues in the liver reached a plateau level of approximately 1 mg/kg (Johnson, 1988).

Monson (1991) analysed, via Raney nickel desulfurization and acid dehydration, the release and characterization of bound carbendazim metabolites in diary cow, goat, hen and rat liver after treatment with $^{14}$C-carbendazim. Using this technique, he was able to show that bound $^{14}$C residue was released from the liver of cows (76% bound before desulfurization and 36% bound after desulfurization) and hens (58% bound before desulfurization and 19% bound after desulfurization). The major part of the reduced residue was identified as 5-HBC, 5,6-HOBC or carbendazim, suggesting that the bound liver residue consisted of conjugates of benzimidazole-related products and not natural products resulting from breakdown and incorporation.

Benomyl and carbendazim are metabolized in fish to 5-HBC (Du Pont, 1972).

## 6.4 Elimination and excretion

Carbendazim is rapidly excreted in the urine and faeces.

In a rat gavage study (Monson, 1990), [phenyl(U)-$^{14}$C]-carbendazim was administered to Sprague-Dawley rats using three dosing regimes: a single oral dose of 50 mg/kg (low dose); a single oral dose of 50 mg/kg following pre-conditioning gavage with unlabelled carbendazim of 50 mg/kg for 14 days (pre-conditioned low dose); and a single oral dose of 1000 mg/kg (high dose). Each dosing group comprised five animals of each sex. A preliminary

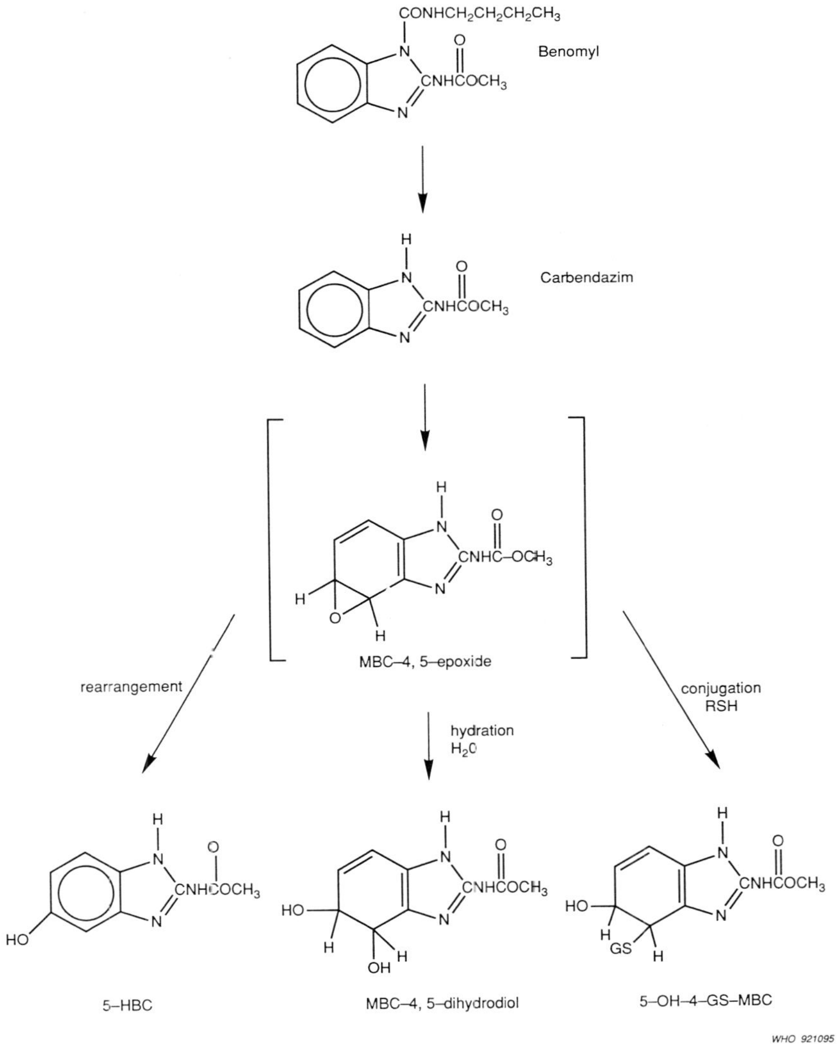


Fig. 2. Proposed metabolic pathway for carbendazim in the laying hen

study conducted with two rats of each sex, each rat having received a single oral dose of 50 mg/kg, demonstrated that 95% of the radioactivity excreted in the urine and faeces was recovered within 72 h after dosing and that < 1% of the dose was expired as volatile metabolites. In the full study, > 98% of the recovered radioactivity was excreted by the time of sacrifice (i.e. 72 h after dosing) in the case of each group of rats. Urinary excretion accounted for 62% to 66% of the dose in males and 54% to 62% of the dose in low-dose and pre-conditioned low-dose females. In the high-dose group, this pathway accounted for 41% of the dose in all animals. Elimination of radiolabel in faeces accounted for virtually all of the remaining radiolabel.

A lactating Holstein cow was dosed by capsule twice daily (483 mg [2-$^{14}$C]-carbendazim each dose), equivalent to 50 mg/kg in the average total daily diet, for five consecutive days, and samples of urine, faeces and milk were collected at each dosing. Five days after the initial dose, 65% of the radiolabel had been excreted in the urine, 21% in the faeces and 0.4% in the milk (a total of 86.4%). Radioactive residues in the urine comprised 48% 5-HBC and 3% polar water-soluble metabolites (Monson, 1985).

In a further study, lactating Holstein cows were dosed by the dietary route with 0, 2, 10 or 50 mg carbendazim/kg diet for 28 days. The highest levels of carbendazim metabolites in the urine and faeces were found in cows fed 50 mg/kg. The highest levels found in urine were 12.56 mg 5-HBC/litre and 1.29 mg 4-HBC per litre. In the faeces 3.81 mg 5-HBC/kg and 0.99 mg carbendazim/kg were detected (but not in the same cow). No carbendazim residues were found in the urine (Hughes, 1984).

Groups of hens were dosed with [2-$^{14}$C]-carbendazim at a rate equivalent to 5 and 120 mg/kg in the average total daily feed for six consecutive days and were sacrificed 24 h after the sixth dose. At sacrifice, an average of 95% and 92% of the radioactive doses had been excreted in the low-dose and high-dose hens, respectively (Monson, 1986).

## 6.5 Reaction with body components

In a study by Guengerich (1981), the effects of carbendazim on hepatic enzyme induction were studied in male and female Crl-CD rats. The treatment groups included animals fed for 28 days with diets that contained carbendazim at concentrations of 0, 10, 30, 100, 300, 1000 or 3000 mg/kg. Microsomal epoxide hydrolase and cytosolic glutathione-*S*-transferase were monitored in subcellular fractions isolated from the livers of animals in each treatment group. Liver weights were also recorded. Elevated liver weights were observed at 1000 and 3000 mg carbendazim/kg in both male and female rats. No apparent liver toxicity or effect on body weight was observed. Carbendazim induced epoxide hydrolase in both sexes of rats and mice at 1000 and 3000 mg/kg. Induction of glutathione-*S*-transferase was observed at 3000 mg/kg. In general, the level of induction seemed to be slightly greater in females than males.

In the same study, but in a separate test, CD-1 male mice were treated via gavage with carbendazim suspended in corn oil (0, 100 and 1000 mg/kg per day) for 5 days. The liver samples were homogenized and subcellular fractions were prepared as above. Wet liver weights, microsomal cytochrome P-450, NADPH-cytochrome-c reductase, styrene-7,8-hydrolase, benzphetamine-*N*-demethylase, benzo(a)pyrene hydroxylase and 7-ethoxycoumarin *O*-deethylase, and cytosolic glutathione-*S*-transferase were measured. Those parameters showing statistically significant increases over the control values were styrene-7,8-hydrolase and glutathione-*S*-transferase; 7-ethoxycoumarin *O*-deethylase showed a significant decrease. It is noteworthy that the total microsomal cytochrome P-450 level did not increase, indicating that a whole scale microsomal induction phenomena was not induced by carbendazim even at the higher treatment level. However, as shown by the increase in microsomal styrene-7,8-hydrolase, some hepatic microsomal enzymes are induced by *in vivo* carbendazim treatment (Guengerich, 1981). There did not appear to be any substantial difference in enzyme induction between rats and mice.

# 7. EFFECTS ON LABORATORY MAMMALS AND *IN VITRO* TEST SYSTEMS

## 7.1 Single exposure

The acute toxicity of carbendazim in several animal species is summarized in Table 8. The $LD_{50}$ values range from > 2000 to > 15 000 mg/kg for a wide variety of test animals and routes of administration. A description of toxic effects is given in section 7.5.1.

## 7.2 Short-term exposure

### 7.2.1 *Gavage*

Groups of ChR-CD male rats (six per dose level) were gavaged with 200, 3400 and 5000 mg carbendazim/kg per day, five times/week, for two weeks. Two out of six rats died at the dose level of 3400 mg/kg per day. At all dose levels, gross and microscopic evidence of adverse effects on testes and reduction or absence of sperm in the epididymides was seen. Testes were small and discoloured, with tubular degeneration and evidence of aspermatogenesis. At the dose level of 3400 mg/kg per day, there were also morphological changes in the duodenum (oedema and focal necrosis), bone marrow (reduction in the blood-forming elements) and liver (decrease in the large globular-shaped vacuoles) (Sherman, 1965; Sherman & Krauss, 1966).

Subchronic administration of 0, 16, 32 or 64 mg carbendazim per kg per day by gavage for 90 days to four groups of 10 male and 10 female litter-mate weaning Wistar rats was carried out. The erythrocyte counts for treated rats were lower than those of the controls after 15 days of exposure. However, no clear dose-response relationship was demonstrated after 30, 60 or 90 days of exposure. A decrease was noted in leucocyte counts at 15 days. After 30 and 60 days, both sexes demonstrated transient decreases in lymphocyte counts compared to controls. However, no clear dose-response relationship was observed among the treated groups. No change was noted in the activity of whole blood cholinesterase. Male rats showed significantly increased alkaline phosphatase activity at a dose level of 64 mg/kg per day. Blood urea levels were lower in males at dose levels of 32 and 64 mg/kg per day

Table 8. Acute toxicity of carbendazim in animals

| Chemical | Species | Sex | Animals per group | Route | Vehicle | Concentration[a] (mg/kg body weight) | Reference |
|---|---|---|---|---|---|---|---|
| Carbendazim (MBC) | rat | M/F | 10 | oral | sesame oil | $LD_{50}$ > 15 000 | Kramer & Weigand (1971) |
| | rat | M | 10 | intraperitoneal | 0.9% saline and Tween 80 | $LD_{50}$ > 2000 | Goodman & Sherman (1974) |
| | rat | M | 6 | inhalation (1 h) | dust | ALC > 5.9 mg/litre[b] | Sarver (1975) |
| | rat | F | 5 | dermal | sesame oil | ALD > 2000 | Kramer & Weigand (1971) |
| | mouse | M | 10 | oral | propylene glycol | $LD_{50}$ > 15 000 | Til & Beems (1981) |
| | mouse | M/F | 10 | intraperitoneal | sesame oil | $LD_{50}$ > 15 000 | Scholz & Weigand (1972) |
| | dog | M/F | 2 | oral | sesame oil | $ALD_{50}$ > 5000 | Scholz & Weigand (1972) |
| | guinea-pig | M | 10 | oral | corn oil | $LD_{50}$ > 5000 | Dashiell (1975) |
| | rabbit | M | 10 | dermal | aqueous paste | $LD_{50}$ > 10 000 | Edwards (1974a) |
| 75% wettable powder | rat | M/F | 5 | oral | corn oil | $LD_{50}$ > 5000 | Hinckle (1981) |
| | rat | M/F | 10 | inhalation | dust | $LC_{50}$ > 5 mg/litre | Nash & Ferenz (1982) |
| | rabbit | M/F | 5 | dermal | physiological saline | $LD_{50}$ > 2000 | Ford (1982) |
| Benlate C (50% wettable powder) | rat | M/F | 5 | oral | water | $LD_{50}$ > 5000 | Grandizio & Sarver (1987) |
| | rabbit | M/F | 5 | dermal | aqueous paste | $LD_{50}$ > 2000 | Vick & Brock (1987b) |

[a] ALC = approximate lethal concentration; ALD = approximate lethal dose
[b] Time-weighted concentration

after 90 days. Increased serum bilirubin concentrations were observed in males and females at 32 and 64 mg/kg per day and were attributable to parenchymal cell damage, as shown by increased glutamic-pyruvic transaminase activity. Dose-related changes in the liver ranged from sparse infiltration by inflammatory cells to inflammatory and degenerative changes. Tubular dilation and hydropic degeneration were noted in the kidneys of the low-dose rats, and fibrosis and congestion in the medium- and high-dose rats. Increased lung weight was correlated with bronchopneumonic changes. Slight changes in weights were reported for several organs (Janardhan et al., 1987). The published information was difficult to evaluate due to the variability of the results and absence of the raw data.

### 7.2.2 *Feeding*

#### 7.2.2.1 *Rat*

Groups of ChR-CD rats (16 males and 16 females per group) were fed carbendazim (72% a.i.) in the diet for 90 days at levels of 0, 100, 500 and 2500 mg/kg. The animals were observed daily for behavioural changes and body weight, and food consumption were recorded at weekly intervals. Haematological examinations were conducted on 10 male and 10 female rats in each group at 30, 60 and 90 days. Routine urinalyses were performed on the same animals, and plasma alkaline phosphatase and glutamic-pyruvic transaminase levels were determined. After 90 to 98 days of continuous feeding, 10 male and 10 female rats in each group were killed and selected organs weighed. These and other organs were preserved for microscopic examination. The six male and six female rats remaining in each group after terminal sacrifice were used in a reproduction study (see section 7.5.1). There were no signs of poisoning and no compound-related effects on weight gain, food consumption or haematological parameters. There were no control data for biochemical determinations, urinalysis or differential white blood counts. The average dose for the high-dose animals was 360 mg/kg per day initially and 123-152 mg/kg per day at sacrifice. The liver-to-body-weight ratio in females fed 2500 mg/kg diet was slightly increased compared with control rats. There were no effects on testicular weights in any of the treatment groups. Microscopic examination of selected tissues and organs in the control and high-dose groups demonstrated no adverse effects attributable to carbendazim (Sherman, 1968).

### 2.2.2 Dog

Groups of one-year-old beagles (four males and four females per group) were administered carbendazim (53% a.i.) in the diet for three months at dietary levels of 0, 100, 500 and 2500 mg/kg. The highest level was reduced to 1500 mg/kg because of reduced food intake and decreased body weight. However, compound administration was interrupted when animals were fed a control diet for a few days and then fed with 1500 mg/kg again.

Food consumption and body weight data were recorded weekly, and clinical laboratory examinations (including haematological, biochemical and urinalysis measurements) were performed pre-test and after 1, 2 and 3 months of feeding. At the end of the study all animals were killed, selected organs were weighed, and these and other organs were subjected to gross and microscopic evaluations.

No mortality or adverse clinical signs were observed over the course of the study, and growth and food consumption were normal (except at 1500-2500 mg/kg). Urinalysis measurements were unaffected by treatment, and there were no dose-related effects on the haematological values. Females at the mid-dose level showed a trend toward increased cholesterol levels at 1, 2 and 3 months compared with the pre-test and control values. High-dose females had similarly elevated cholesterol levels. Organ-to-body weight changes were observed in the case of the thymus of low- and mid-dose males and the prostate of mid-dose males. All the weights for these organs were increased compared with control values. However, only the liver, kidney and testes were examined histologically in the low- and mid-dose groups. Limited histopathological data did not indicate compound-related effects (Sherman, 1970).

In a study by Til et al. (1972), groups of beagles (four males and four females per group) were administered carbendazim in the diet at levels of 0, 100, 300 and 1000 mg/kg for 13 weeks. The highest level was increased to 2000 mg/kg after six weeks of treatment. Body weight, haematological and blood chemistry measurements, urinalyses and liver/kidney function tests were performed periodically. Gross and microscopic examinations of all animals were performed at the end of the study. There were no reported compound-related effects on clinical behaviour, body weight, food consumption, haematological parameters, kidney function (phenol red excretion) or liver function (BSP retention) examinations. Blood chemistry measurements were normal, except for a slight decrease in albumin in mid- and high-dose males at 12 weeks. These values differed from week 0 measurements only in high-dose males. Urinalysis values were normal except for a high bacterial count in high-dose females at week 13. The blood clotting time was slightly reduced in high-dose dogs at week 12. There were slight increases in relative liver and thyroid weights and a decrease in relative heart weights in the highest-dose group compared with controls. No microscopic changes that could be associated with treatment were observed in these or any other organs. Carbendazim appeared to be without adverse effects on beagles when incorporated in the diet for 13 weeks at dietary levels of 300 mg/kg or less.

### 7.2.3 Dermal

New Zealand albino rabbits (six males/group) were treated with 0 or 2000 mg/kg of carbendazim, applied as a 50% aqueous paste to shaved intact dorsal skin. The material was applied repeatedly, 6 h/day, for ten consecutive days. There were no adverse effects on body weight, clinical symptoms, organ weights, gross pathology or histopathology of selected organs. However, there was focal necrosis of the epidermis and polymorphonuclear cell infiltration of the dermis in five out of six exposed rabbits. No other effects were observed (Dashiell, 1975).

## 7.3 Skin and eye irritation; sensitization

### 7.3.1 Dermal

The primary dermal irritation potential of Benlate C (50% wettable powder) was evaluated by applying a 5-g aliquot for 4 h to the clipped intact skin of six New Zealand White rabbits. Test sites were evaluated for erythema, oedema and other evidence of dermal effects, and were scored according to the Draize scale at 4, 24, 48 and 72 h after application. No dermal irritation was seen at any time during the study (Vick & Brock, 1987a).

### 7.3.2 Eye

No eye irritation potential for technical carbendazim was seen in six albino rabbits (Edwards, 1974b). In a study by Vick & Valentine (1987), a 50% wettable powder (formulation) was evaluated for acute eye irritation potential in six male New Zealand white rabbits. The formulation produced slight corneal opacity, mild or moderate conjunctival redness, and slight or mild conjunctival oedema in all the rabbits. In addition, there was moderate iritis in three of the rabbits and minimal blood-tinged discharge in one rabbit. Microscopic examinations revealed no corneal injury in any of the treated eyes. The treated eyes of the two other rabbits were normal by 72 h. It was concluded that this formulation was a moderate eye irritant.

### 7.3.3 Sensitization

Albino guinea-pigs (10 males) exposed to carbendazim, either technical material or a 75% wettable powder formulation, presented no evidence of dermal sensitization following either intradermal injections or repeat applications to shaved intact skin (Ford, 1981).

A 50% carbendazim formulation was tested on the shaved intact skin of 10 male and 10 female Duncan Hartley albino guinea-pigs. Five male and five female guinea-pigs were treated with 80% ethanol (in water) and served as vehicle control animals. Two male and two female guinea-pigs were treated with the test material (as a solid) at the challenge phase only and served as negative control animals. 1-Chloro-2,4-dinitrobenzene (DNCB) was tested as a 0.3% suspension in 80% ethanol (in water) on the shaved intact skin of two male and two female guinea-pigs as a positive control group. No irritation was observed in the test or vehicle control guinea-pigs or in the negative controls at the challenge phase. DNCB produced sensitization in all treated animals (Martin et al., 1987).

## 7.4 Long-term exposure

### 7.4.1 Rat

Groups of weanling rats (36 male and 36 female ChR-CD albino rats/group) were administered carbendazim (50-70% a.i.) in the diet for 104 weeks at levels of 0, 100, 500, 2500 (increased to 10 000 mg/kg after 20 weeks) and 5000 mg/kg diet. Body weight and food consumption were recorded weekly for the first year and twice a month thereafter. Daily observations were made with respect to behavioural changes and mortality. At periodic intervals throughout the study, haematological, urinalysis and selected clinical chemistry examinations were performed. After one year each group was reduced to 30 male and 30 female rats by interim sacrifice for gross and microscopic examinations. At the end of the study all surviving animals were sacrificed and gross examination of tissues and organs was made. Microscopic examinations were conducted on all tissues and organs from the control and 2500-mg/kg groups, the livers of the 100- and 500-mg/kg groups, and the livers, kidneys, testes and bone marrow from the 5000-mg/kg groups. Survival decreased during the second year to approximately 50% for males and 39% for females in all groups. Body weight gain was depressed for males and females in the 2500-mg/kg group and for females in the 5000-mg/kg group, compared to control groups. Food consumption did not differ among the various groups. The average daily dose for the 500-mg/kg group was 65 mg/kg body weight per day initially, 18 mg/kg body weight per day at one year, and 15 mg/kg body weight per day at two years. Haematological examinations demonstrated reduced erythrocyte count and haemoglobin and haematocrit values for females at 9-24 months in the 2500- and 5000-mg/kg groups, and for males at 24 months in the 2500-mg/kg group. There were no compound-related clinical manifestations of toxicity and no effects observed in urinalysis examination. Alkaline phosphatase and glutamic-pyruvic transaminase activity varied throughout the test at 2500 and 5000 mg/kg but did not demonstrate a consistent dose-response relationship. There were no apparent differences in the organ weights or organ-to-body weight measurements, except in the case of female livers in the 2500- and 5000-mg/kg groups. This increase in the liver-to-body weight ratio was due to a reduction in body weight. Histopathological examination of the livers did not demonstrate any compound-related effects. Males in the 2500-mg/kg group presented a marginal increase in diffuse testicular atrophy and prostatitis (Sherman, 1972).

In another 2-year rat study, groups of Wistar rats (60 males and 60 females/group) were administered carbendazim (99% pure) in the diet at levels of 0, 150, 300 and 2000 mg/kg diet for two years. The dose of 2000 mg/kg was increased to 5000 mg/kg after one week and then to 10 000 mg/kg after two weeks for the remainder of the study. Animals were examined daily for clinical signs of toxicity. Body weight and food consumption were measured regularly throughout the study. Haematological (peripheral blood), blood chemistry (orbital sinus) and urinalysis evaluations were conducted periodically during the study. All animals were subjected to complete gross necropsy, and selected organs were weighed. Tissues were examined microscopically in 20 male and 20 female rats in the control and high-dose groups. All tumours and gross abnormalities were also examined histologically. There were no differences between test groups and control animals concerning clinical signs of toxicity or food consumption. Body weights were significantly reduced in low-dose males from week 88 to term and in high-dose females from week 12 to term. Urinalyses were comparable among all groups. Of the haematological parameters examined, haemoglobin was depressed in high-dose females at weeks 26, 52 and 103 and haematocrit was depressed in high-dose females at week 103. There were no compound-related effects in males. Serum glutamic oxaloacetic transaminase (SGOT) activity was decreased in high-dose males at term, but not in females. High-dose females had increased serum glutamic pyruvic transaminase (SGPT) activity and decreased total serum protein at study termination. There were no compound-related effects on organ weights except for increased relative liver weights in high-dose females. There were also no compound-related effects on mortality, this being 50% at week 76 in control males and at week 92 in treated males. There was 50% mortality in control and low-dose females at week 88 and in mid- and high-dose females at 92-96 weeks. Survival at termination of the study was similar in all groups.

There were no histological differences between control and treated groups except for an increased incidence of diffuse proliferation of parafollicular cells of the thyroid in the high-dose females (Til et al., 1976a).

### 7.4.2 Dog

In a one-year study, beagle dogs (five of each sex per group) were fed diets containing 0, 100, 200 or 500 mg carbendazim/kg. The dogs were weighed at regular intervals, and individual food consumption was monitored throughout the study. Clinical pathology evaluations were performed twice prior to the initiation of the study and five times during the study, at 1, 3, 6, 9 and 12 months. After one year, all dogs were killed and selected tissues were examined microscopically. There were no statistical differences in mean body weight that could be attributed to carbendazim exposure. The mean daily food consumption in all treated groups of dogs was similar to controls. None of the clinical observations were attributable to carbendazim intake. Dogs fed 500 mg/kg had elevated levels of serum cholesterol. These levels were statistically significant for the males at 9 months and the females at 1 and 2 months. There were no compound-related microscopic lesions related to carbendazim intake (Stadler, 1986).

Groups of beagles (four males and four females per group) were administered carbendazim (53% a.i.) in the diet at dosage levels of 0, 100, 500 and 2500 mg/kg for two years. The dogs were 1-2 years of age at the start of the test. Food consumption and body weight data were obtained weekly and animals were examined daily for clinical signs of toxicity. Haematological, biochemical and urinalysis examinations were performed periodically throughout the study. Interim sacrifice after one year was performed on one male and one female from the control and 500-mg/kg groups. Organ weight, gross necropsy and histopathological examinations were performed at the end of the study. Only the livers and testes were examined histologically in the 100- and 500-mg/kg groups. No mortality was reported for the control or the 100- and 500-mg/kg dose groups. The average daily intake for the 500-mg/kg dose group was 15.0-20 mg/kg body weight per day initially, 14-18 mg/kg body weight per day after one year and 10-16 mg/kg body weight per day after two years. Haematological and urinalysis values were unaffected by treatment. The dogs in the 500-mg/kg groups had increased levels of cholesterol, blood urea nitrogen (BUN), total protein and SGPT. Swollen vacuolated hepatic cells and marginal proliferation of the portal triads with cellular infiltration was observed in one dog sacrificed after one year, which had been fed 500 mg/kg. No histopathological liver lesions were observed in animals fed 500 mg/kg diet at the end of the study. Although inflammatory and fibrotic liver changes were observed in the 2500-mg/kg group, these changes cannot be evaluated because of the uncertainty of the dosing regime, of the time of exposure and of the number of dogs. There were no noticeable effects on organ weights or on organ-to-body weight ratios. Diffuse testicular atrophy and aspermatogenesis were observed in males (two out of four) at 100 mg/kg but not at 500 mg/kg (Sherman, 1972).

In another 2-year dog study, groups of beagles (four males and four females per group) were fed technical carbendazim in the diet at dosage levels of 0, 150, 300 and 2000 mg/kg for 104 weeks. After 33 weeks the dose 2000 mg/kg was increased to 5000 mg/kg. The dogs were 22-27 weeks old at the start of the study. Daily examinations were made for clinical signs of poisoning or adverse behaviour. Body weight and food consumption data were recorded regularly throughout the study. At periodic intervals (weeks 13, 26, 52, 78 and 104), haematological, blood chemistry and urinalysis measurements were made. Liver function (BSP retention) and kidney function (phenol red excretion) tests were conducted at weeks 26, 52 and 104. At the conclusion of the 104 weeks of dietary administration, each dog was sacrificed and gross and microscopic examination of tissues and organs was performed. There was no mortality in any group except for one female in the high-dose group which was killed in a moribund state after week 36. Body weight was decreased in mid-dose males and high-dose males and females. Food consumption was comparable among all groups. Blood clotting times were significantly reduced in high-dose males from week 13 to term, and slight decreases were noted in high-dose females. Serum alkaline phosphatase activity was increased in the high-dose group throughout the study. There were no compound-related effects on SGPT or SGOT levels. All other haematological and blood chemistry values were comparable with control groups. There were no differences for BSP retention, phenol red excretion or urine analysis values among the various groups. Absolute liver and thyroid weights were significantly increased in high-dose dogs. Relative liver, thyroid and pituitary weights were also significantly increased at the high-dose level. There were no reported microscopic changes in these organs related to treatment. There was an increased incidence of prostatitis (3/4 versus 1/4) in high-dose males compared with controls. Also noted in high-dose males (1/4) was interstitial mononuclear inflammatory cell infiltrates and atrophic tubules of the testes. It was concluded that the feeding of carbendazim in the diet to dogs for two years was without apparent adverse effects at levels up to and including 300 mg/kg (Reuzel et al., 1976).

### 7.4.3 Mouse

A description of studies on mice is given in section 7.7.

## 7.5 Reproduction, embryotoxicity and teratogenicity

### 7.5.1 Reproduction

Groups of ChR-CD rats (3 male and 16 female rats per group, except that the high-dose group contained 20 females) were fed carbendazim in the diet at dose levels of 0, 100, 500, 5000 and 10 000 mg/kg and subjected to a standard two-litter-per-generation, three-generation reproduction study. The parental animals were fed the experimental diet at 21 days of age and mated to produce the $F_1$ litter at 100 days of age. The number of matings, pregnancies and number of young in each litter at birth was recorded. The litters were culled to 10 pups/litter on day 4. The number of the live pups was recorded on days 4, 12 and 21, as was pup weight at weaning. The parents were mated again to produce the $F_{1B}$ litters. The $F_{1B}$ litters were maintained on the respective diets for 110 days and then mated to produce the $F_{2A}$ and $F_{2B}$ litters. The $F_{3A}$ and $F_{3B}$ litters were produced similarly. Gross and histopathological examinations of selected tissues and organs were performed on two males and two females in each of five $F_{3B}$ litters from the control, 5000- and 10 000-mg/kg groups. Reproduction indices, including mating, fecundity, fertility, gestation, viability and lactation, were calculated and compared with control values. Carbendazim was without effect on fertility, gestation, viability and lactation. However, the average litter weights at weaning were reduced in all generations fed 5000 and 10 000 mg/kg. Histopathological examination of $F_{3B}$ weanlings did not reveal any effects that were considered compound-related (Sherman, 1972).

Two additional feeding studies (Sherman, 1968; Koeter et al., 1976) were reviewed by the 1983 Joint FAO/WHO Meeting on Pesticide Residues (JMPR), which concluded that both reports had limitations. For the Sherman (1968) study, it was stated that the "data presented were extremely limited and submitted as group data only. There were no pregnancies at 100 mg/kg diet for either $F_{1a}$ or $F_{1b}$ matings. There were no apparent effects on the reproduction indices on weanling weights. However, the fertility index for all groups, which was 33-67% prevents any meaningful interpretation of the data" (FAO/WHO, 1985b). For the study of Koeter et al. (1976), the 1983 JMPR concluded that "although there were no apparent adverse effects on reproduction and no teratogenic effects at dietary levels of carbendazim up to and including 2000 mg/kg, there were no individual animal data presented. Histopathology of animals in the four-week study was incomplete and did not include evaluations of spleen or ovaries. Such additional data are needed to confirm the absence of adverse effects in this three-generation reproduction study in rats" (FAO/WHO, 1985b).

A serial breeding technique was used to evaluate the fertility of male Sprague-Dawley rats after exposure by gavage to 10 daily doses of carbendazim (400 mg/kg per day). Proven-fertile males (90 days old) were bred with a new female each week. Breeding began on the third day of treatment and continued for 32 weeks after the last day of chemical exposure. Twelve days after each breeding period, the females were killed, their uteri were examined for resorptions, and the number of dead and viable fetuses was determined. All males were killed 35 weeks after the exposure, and testicular tissue was prepared for histopathological examination by vascular perfusion. The fertility (as indicated by the number of pregnant females) of males in the carbendazim-treated group was depressed during the first post-exposure week; 10 of the 24 treated males failed to induce a pregnancy, as compared with no failure in the control group. By the fifth post-exposure week, 16 of the 24 carbendazim-treated males were infertile. Of these 16 males, 4 recovered fertility after being infertile for 5-11 consecutive breeding periods. However, 12 of the males did not recover fertility during the remainder of the 32 week post-exposure period. Histological examinations of testicular sections 245 days after the exposure revealed that the exposure to carbendazim had caused severe seminiferous tubular atrophy (> 85% of tubules were atrophic) in those treated males that failed to recover fertility. The seminiferous tubules of these males often showed "Sertoli cell only" syndrome epithelium surrounded by a thickened basement membrane. Less than 2% of the tubules contained spermatozoa in the lumen. The seminiferous tubules of the carbendazim-treated males that recovered fertility had various numbers of atrophic tubules (13-85%) 245 days after the exposure (Carter et al., 1987).

In another study, groups of male and female rats (8-12 of each sex per group) were administered 0, 50, 100, 200 or 400 mg carbendazim/kg per day by gavage from weaning through puberty, gestation and lactation, and they were mated at 84 days of age. The male rats were killed on day 104-106 while the female rats were killed on day 27 postpartum. A similar study was conducted with Syrian hamsters administered 0 or 400 mg/kg per day. In the parental generation, various landmarks of puberty were measured. In females, estrous cyclicity, litter size, the number of implants, organ weights and histological status were assessed. In males, organ weights, testicular and epididymal sperm counts, sperm motility, sperm morphology, testicular histological status, and endocrine parameters were assessed. In addition, the growth, viability and reproductive function of the offspring ($F_1$) were observed during a 4-month period of continuous breeding. Males were killed at 5 months for histopathological investigation. In the parental generation of both species, carbendazim did not alter pubertal development, growth or viability. The reproductive potential of rats treated with carbendazim with 200 and 400 mg/kg per day was reduced due to effects on sperm production and fetal viability. In the male rat, carbendazim treatment with 200 or 400 mg/kg per day markedly altered sperm morphology, testicular and epididymal weights, sperm numbers and testicular histology. Fertility, sperm motility and hormonal levels were altered primarily in those males fed 200 or 400 mg/kg per day that exhibited very low sperm counts. A statistically significant reduction in caudal epididymal sperm count was noted at dose levels of 50 mg/kg per day or more. Testicular and epididymal sperm counts in male hamsters were significantly lower (about 21%) in the carbendazim-treated males compared with the control males. In the $F_1$ male hamsters, testis and seminal vesicle weights and epididymal sperm counts were significantly reduced by prenatal exposure to carbendazim at 400 mg/kg per day. In the parental female rats, carbendazim administration caused postimplantation losses at 400 mg/kg per day and a few malformed rat pups were found in litters at 100 and 200 mg/kg per day. Litter size was significantly reduced at 200 and 400 mg/kg per day. Overall, carbendazim was less toxic to the hamster than to the rat (Gray et al., 1988, 1990).

Since spermatogenesis is an androgen-dependent process, the effects of carbendazim (0-400 mg/kg per day by gavage) on the endocrine function of the rat testes were investigated. Following subchronic (85 day) exposure, serum hormone levels, including those of pituitary luteinizing hormone (LH), follicle-stimulating hormone (FSH), thyroid-stimulating hormone (TSH), prolactin (PRL), and androgen-binding protein (ABP) and testosterone in testicular fluids (interstitial fluid and seminiferous tubule fluid) were measured. In addition, the functional capacity of the Leydig cell to secrete testosterone was assessed *in vitro* following human chorionic gonadotrophin (HCG) challenge. Subchronic treatment with carbendazim at doses of 50-100 mg/kg per day had no effect on pituitary or testicular hormone concentrations; dosing with 200 mg/kg per day elevated the testosterone concentration in the seminiferous tubule fluid and the ABP tubule fluid without affecting serum testosterone or ABP concentrations. The dose of 400 mg/kg per day resulted in increased concentrations of both testosterone and ABP in the interstitial fluid and seminiferous tubule fluid and of serum ABP, but no change in serum testosterone level. These hormonal changes are consistent with carbendazim effects on the gonads and resultant testicular atrophy. This endocrine profile is similar to the "Sertoli cell only" syndrome discussed by de Krester (1977). Thus, the elevated seminiferous tubule fluid testosterone concentrations may be a result of two factors: (a) greater release of testosterone by the Leydig cells into the interstitial fluid; and/or (b) decreased testosterone outflow from the testis into the general circulation. In addition, increased ABP in the interstitial fluid may reflect a change in the relative secretion of ABP into the interstitial fluid and the seminiferous tubules (Rehnberg et al., 1989).

Since it is possible that extragonadal changes contributed to the appearance of the altered testicular endocrine profile described above, a further study focused on the presence of concurrent changes in the hypothalamus and pituitary control of the testes. In this study, rats were gavaged with carbendazim (50, 100, 200 or 400 mg/kg per day) for 85 days (Gray et al., 1988). A dose-related increase in serum FSH and LH was noted, but values for prolactin and thyroid-stimulating hormone remained unchanged. No statistical differences in gonadotropin-releasing hormone (GnRH) concentrations were present in the mediobasal hypothalamus, although an elevation in anterior hypothalamic GnRH values was found at the 50-mg/kg dose, followed by a dose-related decline. These findings would suggest that carbendazim-induced testicular damage is accompanied by compensatory changes in the hypothalmic and pituitary regulation of the testes (Goldman et al., 1989).

The above studies imply that carbendazim acts directly on the testes to produce a number of hormonal and pathological changes. Consistent with this hypothesis are the results of the study of Nakai et al. (1992), in which the effects of carbendazim on the testes, efferent ductules and spermatozoa were determined after a single oral dose in male Sprague-Dawley rats (Charles Rivers). In the first experiment, groups of 86-day-old rats were treated with 0 or 400 mg carbendazim/kg and killed 2, 4 or 8 h later on the same day or 1, 4, 8, 16 or 32 days after dosing. The effect of carbendazim was first noted at 8 h as an increase in testicular weight. Testis weight continued to increase until day 4 and declined thereafter. On days 16 and 32, testes weights were substantially lower than those of controls in 5 out of 16 animals, indicating the variable response of individual animals. A decrease in the percentage of sonication-resistant sperm heads per testis occurred at 8 h (4 out of 8 rats affected), but this decrease was not significant until 24 h, when a mean decrease of 19% was observed. Maximum decreases in total sperm head counts per testis occurred on day 8, after which some recovery was apparent. Epididymal weights were increased on day 4. The percentage of morphologically normal sperm in the cauda epididymus was less on day 4. By day 8, many spermatozoa heads were separated from their flagella and 10% of the heads were misshapen. Numerous sloughed round germ cells and cytoplasmic testicular debris were also evident. No effect on the percentage of motile sperm was seen at 2, 4 and 8 h or at 1 and 4 days post-treatment. Sperm motility was significantly decreased on days 8 and 16. Because of the clumping and degeneration of the spermatozoa, quantitative estimates of the percentage motility could not be determined on days 8 and 16. Similarly damaged sperm were seen in 3 out of 8 rats on day 32, although the percentage of motile sperm that could be measured was similar to that of controls.

In a second experiment by Nakai et al. (1992), groups of rats (between 97 and 105 days of age) were treated with a single oral dose of 0, 50, 100, 200, 400 or 800 mg/kg and killed on day 2 or 70 post-treatment. On day 2, a dose-dependent increase in testicular weight was seen at dose levels 100 mg/kg or more. This was accompanied by significant increases in mean seminiferous tubular diameter at 400 and 800 mg/kg. At 50 mg/kg, missing immature germ cells were noted with round spermatids from stages I and II and elongated spermatids sloughed from stage VII epithelium. At 100 mg/kg, the disappearance of germ cells was more severe and sloughing of elongated spermatids extended into stages XII and XIV. A detailed description of the spermatogenic cycle may be found in Russell et al. (1990). At doses higher than 100 mg/kg, missing germ cells extended into all stages except stages IX-XI, while, at doses of 400-800 mg/kg, some seminiferous epithelia were damaged so severely that it was difficult to identify the stage. In addition, major pathological changes were seen in the excurrent ducts of the testis. The rete testis was swollen with sloughed germ cells indicating that ductal blockage had occurred further down the tract. Such occlusions were observed in the efferent ductules of animals treated with 100 mg/kg or more. On day 70, mean testis weight and mean seminiferous tubule diameter showed a dose-dependent decrease. Histologically, these decreases were associated with a dose-dependent increase in seminiferous tubular atrophy. No atrophic tubules were seen in the control rats. The atrophied tubules contained primarily Sertoli cells and occasional spermatogonia, and were surrounded by a thickened basement membrane. Pathological alterations were also seen in the efferent ductules of the treated animals, 50% or more of the ducts being occluded in rats dosed with 100 mg or more. The occlusions were characterized as compacted luminal contents, spermatic granulomas, mineralizations and obliteration of the original lumen by fibrotic connective tissue (Nakai et al., 1992).

In a further study, carbendazim was administered to female Holtzmann rats (8 rats per group) by gavage (0, 25, 50, 100, 200, 400 or 1000 mg/kg per day) during early pregnancy (days 1 to 8). A range of maternal parameters, including the number of implantation sites, body weight gain, uterine weight, implantation site size, and serum ovarian and pituitary hormones, was assessed following sacrifice at day 9. At dosages up to 400 mg/kg per day, carbendazim had no significant effect on any of the measured parameters but a trend towards increased resorptions was evident. The highest dosage produced reductions in maternal body weight gain, implantation site weight and serum LH, and an increase in serum estradiol (Cummings et al., 1990).

Female hamsters were treated with a single gavage dose of carbendazim to identify effects of this compound during the perifertilization period. The exposure times were selected to coincide with either of the two microtubule-dependent events initiated by the ovulatory surge of LH, i.e. oocyte maturation (first meiotic division, occurring late on vaginal proestrous) or fertilization (second meiotic division, occurring early on vaginal estrous). In the first experiment, 0, 250, 500, 750 or 1000 mg carbendazim per kg (10 hamsters per group) was administered during meiosis I. Pregnancy outcome was assessed on day 15. The percentage of pregnant hamsters was significantly reduced at 750 and 1000 mg/kg. In those animals that became pregnant, the average number of live pups was reduced at all dose rates. In a second experiment, female hamsters (10 hamsters per group) were bred overnight and administered a single dose of 0 or 1000 mg/kg during meiosis II on the morning following breeding. The percentage of pregnant hamsters was unaffected, but the average number of live pups (measured at 15 days) was reduced. These results show that carbendazim administration by gavage at microtubule-dependent meiotic events can result in early pregnancy loss in hamsters (Perreault et al., 1992).

In a separate study, pseudopregnant rats (induced by stimulation of the uterine cervix with a small brass rod on proestrous and estrous) were administered 0 or 400 mg carbendazim/kg per day during days 1-8. On day 4 of pseudopregnancy, a uterine decidual cell response was induced and the females were killed on day 9. The decidual cell response, evaluated as a measure of uterine competency, was significantly less in the treated rats than in the controls (Cummings et al., 1990).

Groups of male mice (12 per group) were administered carbendazim (0, 250, 500 or 1000 mg/kg per day) by gavage for 5 consecutive days. Body weights, testis weights and sperm parameters were measured at 7, 24 and 39 days post-treatment. Body weights were unaffected. Testis weights were reduced only in the highest-dose group at 7 and 24 days but had recovered by 39 days. Flow cytometry measurements of testicular cells showed that the relative percentages of certain testicular populations (round, elongating and elongated spermatids) at the highest-dose group were different from the control pattern 7 and 24 day after treatment (Evenson et al., 1987).

### 7.5.2 Embryotoxicity and teratogenicity

Carbendazim (95% purity) was administered by gavage to female Holtzman rats at dose levels of 0, 100, 200, 400 or 600 mg/kg body weight per day during days 1-8 of gestation, and the rats were then sacrificed on days 11 or 20. Maternal toxicity was not observed at any dose level. At day 11, the crown-rump length, head length, number of somites and number of embryos per dam were significantly reduced in groups receiving dosages of 200 mg/kg body weight per day or more. Open posterior neuropores and limb anomalies were observed more frequently at dosages equal to or greater than 200 mg/kg body weight per day. At day 20, increased resorptions, decreased live litter size and fetal body weight and delayed ossification was observed at all dosages. Skeletal malformations at the high dosage levels were attributed to carbendazim exposure. The authors noted that developmental alterations occurred at stages after the termination of dosing, suggesting that either the anomalies represent delays in development or the embryonic cells are vulnerable at earlier stages than was previously thought (Cummings et al., 1992).

Carbendazim, in a 0.5% aqueous suspension of methyl cellulose, was administered by gavage to Crl:CDBR rats (25/dose group) on days 7-16 of gestation at daily doses of 0, 5, 10, 20 or 90 mg/kg per day. Maternal toxicity was seen only at the highest dosage in the form of depressed weight gains during the dosing periods and prior to sacrifice on day 22. Mean values for liver weight and liver-to-body weight ratio were increased. Decreased pregnancy rate was observed at the highest dosage. An increase in the incidence of early resorptions per dam, decreased litter size, and the total resorption of three litters occurred at the highest dosage, only the reduction in females per litter being significant. Significant reductions in mean fetal weight were observed at both 20 and 90 mg/kg per day. A significant increase in the incidence of fetal malformations was also seen at 90 mg/kg per day. The malformations consisted primarily of hydrocephaly, microphthalmia, anophthalmia, malformed scapulae and axial skeletal malformations (vertebral, rib and sternebral fusions, exencephaly, hemivertebrae and rib hyperplasia) (Alverez, 1987). The no-observed-effect levels (NOEL) for the dam and fetus were 20 and 10 mg/kg per day, respectively.

In a further study, Delatour & Besse (1990) reported embryotoxic effects in eleven Sprague-Dawley rats administered 19.1 mg carbendazim/kg per day by gavage from days 8 to 15 of gestation and sacrificed at day 21. The authors reported statistically significant ($P < 0.05$) increases in dead fetuses and fetal skeletal and external malformations, and a statistically significant decrease in fetal weight in the treated group. Since only one dose was used, it was not possible to determine a NOEL.

The effects of carbendazim on fetal survival and development were studied by Janardhan et al. (1984) in rats and rabbits. Female Wistar-rats (8-10 per group) were given carbendazim (98% purity) by gavage (0, 20, 40 and 80 mg/kg per day) on days 6 to 15 of pregnancy. Half of each group of animals was killed on day 21 of gestation and half was allowed to deliver normally. Female albino rabbits were given 0, 40, 80 and 160 mg carbendazim/kg per day by gavage on days 6 to 18 of pregnancy and were sacrificed on day 31. All sacrificed animals were scored for live and dead fetuses and for resorptions; live fetuses were killed and examined for abnormalities. After normal deliveries, neonatal deaths and survivors were counted; survivors were weighed and examined for gross abnormalities. In rats sacrificed on day 21, dead and resorbed fetuses accounted for 29% of conceptuses in controls, 48% at a dosage of 20 mg/kg per day, and 54 to 73% at dosages of 40 and 80 mg/kg per day. In rabbits, dead and resorbed fetuses formed 0% of total conceptuses in controls and 15, 21.7 and 33.3% at 40, 80 and 160 mg/kg per day, respectively. There were no differences among the various groups of rats or rabbits with respect to mean weight of live fetuses, and there were no malformations. In rats giving birth, the average number of live pups per litter was close to 8 in controls, 6 at 20 mg/kg per day, and about 5 at 40 and 80 mg/kg per day. Mean fetal weight was increased by about 13% over controls at the two highest dosages. There were no still births, neonatal deaths or gross abnormalities, but mortality at 21 days postpartum was 3.0 to 3.5 times greater at the two highest-doses compared to control (Janardhan et al., 1984).

Suspensions of carbendazim (in aqueous 0.5% carboxymethylcellulose) were administered by gavage on days 7 to 19 of presumed gestation to artificially inseminated New Zealand white rabbits (20 rabbits per group). Dose levels were 0, 10, 20 and 125 mg/kg per day (based on active ingredient) in a volume of 5 ml/kg. The administration of 125 mg/kg per day inhibited average maternal weight until day 16 of gestation. There was a slightly decreased implantation rate at 20 and 125 mg/kg per day and an increased incidence of resorption at 125 mg/kg per day. These effects resulted in a decreased live litter size at these two dosages. At 125 mg/kg per day, litters showed decreased fetal body weight, but the effect was not statistically significant. The average percentage of malformed fetuses per litter was significantly increased at 125 mg/kg per day. Compound-related malformations at the highest dosage consisted of malformed cervical vertebrae and interrelated malformation of the ribs and proximate thoracic vertebrae (Christian et al., 1985). The NOEL for maternal toxicity was 20 mg/kg per day and the NOEL for developmental toxicity was 10 mg/kg per day.

Groups of ChR-CD rats (27-28 pregnant rats per group) were administered carbendazim (53% a.i.) in their diet at levels of 0, 100, 500, 2500, 5000, 7500 and 10 000 mg/kg from day 6 to day 15 of gestation. Average doses were equivalent to 0, 8.9, 45.9, 218.4, 431.6, 625.5 and 746.9 mg/kg body weight per day, respectively. On day 20 of gestation, all pregnant animals were sacrificed and fetuses delivered by Caesarean section. There was no mortality, no adverse effect on body weight or clinical signs of toxicity. Food intake was reduced at the highest-dose level during the period the test diet was administered, but returned to control levels from days 16 to 20. The number of implantation sites, resorption sites and live/dead fetuses were not adversely affected by carbendazim (Sherman, 1970). After evaluating this study, the 1983 JMPR concluded that there were no external or internal abnormalities reported that could be considered compound-related. However, no individual litter data were presented (FAO/WHO, 1985b).

In a further study (Koeter, 1975a), pregnant Wistar-SPF rats (18-22 per group) were administered carbendazim in the diet at dosage levels of 0, 600, 2000 and 6000 mg/kg from days 6 to 15 of gestation. No individual animal or litter data were reported, and variations in ossification and other skeletal abnormalities were presented as percentages. Therefore, the teratogenic or fetotoxic potential of carbendazim to pregnant Wistar-SPF rats cannot be determined from the results and data presented (FAO/WHO, 1985b).

Groups of pregnant New Zealand albino rabbits (3-11 per group) were administered carbendazim in the diet at dosage levels of 0, 600, 2000 and 6000 mg/kg from day 6 to 18 of gestation (Koeter, 1975b). There was a significant increase in the number of supernumery ribs (bilateral) and skull bones in the highest-dose group and ossification was significantly delayed or absent in these fetuses. However, there were no individual animal or litter data, variations in ossification were presented as percentages, and visceral anomalies were evaluated in only two of the four groups. The teratogenic potential of carbendazim to pregnant New Zealand albino rabbits, therefore, cannot be ascertained from the results and data presented (FAO/WHO, 1985b).

## 7.6 Mutagenicity and related end-points

Numerous studies have been conducted to assess the mutagenic potential of carbendazim. Many of the results are conflicting and many of the study reports do not provide sufficient detail to evaluate the reasons for the conflicting data. Prior to the mid-1980s, industrially produced carbendazim contained phenazine impurities. Therefore, different degrees of purity of carbendazim might account for some of the discrepancies. Table 9 presents those studies that reported sufficient experimental detail and data.

Carbendazim is not a heritable gene mutagen. It does not interact with cellular DNA, induce point mutations or result in germ cell mutations. This has been demonstrated in both mammalian and non-mammalian systems *in vitro* and *in vivo*, and in somatic cells as well as in germ cells. Positive results have occasionally been obtained in gene mutation studies, but this was due to the presence of phenazines. These contaminants are mutagenic at very low concentrations in the *Salmonella typhimurium* Ames test and also in the mouse lymphoma Y5178Y $TK^{+/-}$ gene mutation assay. Concentrations of > 4 mg diaminophenazine/kg and 10 mg aminohydroxyphenazine/kg resulted in positive *Salmonella typhimurium* Ames test results. Process changes by some of the major carbendazim manufacturers have removed the phenazines. This contaminant is not present when other benzimidazoles such as benomyl or thiophanate-methyl are metabolized to carbendazim. Carbendazim does cause numerical chromosome aberrations (aneuploidy and/or polyploidy) in experimental systems *in vitro* and *in vivo*.

## 7.7 Carcinogenicity

In a study by Wood (1982), groups of CD-1 mice (80 males and 80 females per group) were administered carbendazim (99% a.i.) in the diet at dose levels of 0, 500, 1500 and 7500 mg/kg diet for two years. The highest-dose was reduced to 3750 mg/kg after

Table 9. Studies on mutagenicity of carbendazim

| End-points/Tests | Species, strains | Concentration | Activation | Result | Reference |
|---|---|---|---|---|---|
| **1. DNA damage and repair** | | | | | |
| | *Bacillus subtilis* | 20-1000 μg per disk | without | negative | Shirasu et al. (1977) |
| | *Salmonella typhimurium* (TA1535, TA1938) | 125-2000 μg/plate | NR | negative | Rashid & Mumma (1986) |
| | *Escherichia Coli*, K-12 | 125-2000 μg/plate | NR | | |
| | *E. Coli*, WP2 | 125-2000 μg/plate | NR | negative | |
| Sister chromatid exchanges | CHO cells | 0.13-40.0 μg/ml | without | negative | Ivett (1984) |
| | | 1.25-40.0 μg/ml | with | negative | |
| Sister chromatid exchanges | human lymphocytes | 0.03-30.0 μg/ml | with and without | negative | Banduhn & Obe (1985) |
| Sister chromatid exchanges | human lymphocytes | 1-60 μg/ml (technical grade) | with and without | marginal positive at 30 μg/ml and above | Pandita (1988) |

Table 9 (contd).

| | | | | | |
|---|---|---|---|---|---|
| Unscheduled DNA synthesis | male mouse hepatocytes | 0.125-12.5 μg/ml | | | Tong (1981a,b) |
| | male rat hepatocytes | 0.0125-12.5 μg/ml | | | |
| Unscheduled DNA synthesis | rat hepatocytes | 1.04-104.0 μg/ml | | negative | Litton (1981) |
| **2. Gene mutation** | | | | | |
| (1) Bacterial gene mutation assays | *S. typhimurium*, TA1535, TA1537, TA98, TA100 | 4-2500 μg/plate | with and without | negative | Gericke (1977) |
| Overlay spot test | *S. typhimurium, his* G46, TA1530, TA1950 | 50-100 μg/spot | | weak mutagenic activity at 100 μg/spot | Fiscor et al. (1978) |
| Plate incorporation assay | TA100 | 50-200 μg/plate | NR | negative | Fiscor et al. (1978) |
| Spot, liquid culture & host mediated assays | *S. typhimurium, his* G46, TA1530, TA1535, TA1950 | 0.25-10 000 μg/ml | | negative | Fiscor et al. (1978) |
| Plate incorporation assay | *S. typhimurium* (TA1535, TA1537, TA1538, TA100) | 5-1000 μg/plate | with and without | negative | Shirasu et al. (1977) |
| | *E. coli*, WP2 *hcr* | 5-1000 μg/plate | with and without | negative | Shirasu et al. (1977) |

Table 9 (contd).

| End-points/Tests | Species, strains | Concentration | Activation | Result | Reference |
|---|---|---|---|---|---|
| | *S. typhimurium* (TA98, TA100) | 1-300 µg/plate | with and without | negative | Pandita (1988) |
| | *S. typhimurium* (TA1537, TA1538, TA97, TA98) | 5000 µg/plate | | positive in TA1537 & TA97 (using a pre-incubation assay), positive in TA1538 & TA98 only with activation | Albertini (1989) |
| | *S. typhimurium* (TA1535, TA1537, TA98, TA100) | 100-10 000[a] µg per plate | with and without | positve at 5000 µg/plate with activation in TA98, TA1537 | Donovan (1982) |
| | *S. typhimurium* (TA1535, TA1537, TA98, TA100) | up to 10 000[b] µg per plate | with and without | negative up to 10 000 µg/plate | Russell (1983) |
| | *S. typhimurium* | | | positive if carbendazim samples with 4 ppm DAP or 10 ppm AHP impurities | Arce (1984a,b) |

Table 9 (contd).

| | | | | | |
|---|---|---|---|---|---|
| Host mediated assay | male ICR mice<br>*S. typhimurium his* G46 | Total dose of mice<br>1000, 4000 mg/kg | | negative | Shirasu et al. (1977) |
| | *S. typhimurium* (TA1535, TA1537, TA98, TA100) | 2-AB<br>100-10 000 µg/plate | with and without | negative | Donovan (1983); Russell (1977) |
| | | 5-HBC 200-20000 µg/plate | | negative | |
| (2) Yeast & fungal mutation assays | *A. nidulans* | 2.77 µM<br>(0.53 µg/ml) | without | increase in frequency of colonies resistant to carbendazim | Speakman & Nirenberg (1981) |
| | *Cladosporium cucumerinum* | 0.58 µM<br>(0.11 µg/ml) | without | no effect on frequency of colonies resistant to carbendazim | Speakman & Nirenberg (1981) |
| | *Saccharomyces cerevisiae* D7 | 10-40 µg/ml | | negative | Albertini (1991) |
| (3) *In vitro* gene mutation assays | | | | | |
| HGPRT | CHO cells | 3-628 µM<br>3-654 µM | with<br>without | negative | Waterer (1980) |

Table 9 (contd).

| End-points/Tests | Species, strains | Concentration | Activation | Result | Reference |
|---|---|---|---|---|---|
| forward mutation at TK locus | mouse L5178Y lymphoma cells | 50-250 μM | with and without | positive with activation at 100 μM, negative without activation | Jotz (1980) |
| (4) Insect germ cell gene mutation | | | | | |
| Sex-linked recessive lethals | *Drosophila melanogaster* | 0.5 mg/ml in DMSO | | negative | Lamb & Lilly (1980) |
| Germline aneuploidy | *D. melanogaster*, FIX, ZESTE | 400-50 000 ppm feeding to larvae or young adult females | | negative | Osgood et al. (1991) |
| (5) *In vivo* mammalian gene mutation assays | mouse embryos treated *in utero* by dosing the mother 100-300 mg/kg orally | | | 200 mg/kg positive | Fahrig & Seiler (1979) |
| **3. Chromosomal effects** | | | | | |
| (1) *In vitro* chromosomal effect | *S. cerevisiae* | 0.001-0.100 mg/ml | | maximum responses for mitotic & meiotic chromosome gain at 0.05 and 0.025 mg/ml | Whittaker et al. (1990) |

Table 9 (contd).

| | | | | | |
|---|---|---|---|---|---|
| | *S. cerevisiae* | 5 $\mu$g/ml | | positive for aneuploidy | Albertini (1991) |
| | human lymphocytes | 0.1-10.0 $\mu$M | with and without | not clastogenic, but induce micro-nuclei at $\geq$ 10 $\mu$M | Danduhn & Obe (1985) |
| | human lymphocytes | 0.5 mg/ml | without | did not increase chromosome aberr-ation frequency | Lamb & Lilly (1980) |
| (2) *In vivo* mammalian chromosomal effect | | | | | |
| | male & female Sprague-Dawley rat bone marrow cells | single oral dose 300 mg/kg | | did not increase chromosome aberr-ation frequency | BASF (1975); FAO/WHO (1985b) |
| | Chinese hamster bone marrow cells | oral, 1000 mg/kg | | did not produce chromosome breakage | Seiler (1976) |
| | ICR mice nucleated anaphase cells | 2 oral dose of 1000 mg/kg | | exhibit lagging chro-mosome, bridge for-mation, tripolar spindle formation, etc | Seiler (1976) |

Table 9 (contd).

| End-points/Tests | Species, strains | Concentration | Activation | Result | Reference |
|---|---|---|---|---|---|
| | Mouse bone marrow | 500 mg/kg | | did not detect micronuclei | Seiler (1976) |
| | Swiss albino mice | 0, 200, 1000, 2000, 4000 or 6000 mg/kg i.p. | | dose dependent increase in micronucleus | Pandita (1988) |
| | male Chinese hamsters bone marrow | 0, 100, 500 or 1000 mg/kg i.p. | | no effect on hyperploidy | Pandita (1988) |
| (3) *In vivo* germ cell chromosomal mutation | | | | | |
| Mouse dominant lethal test | NMRI mice | 500 mg/kg i.p. per day, 5 days | | did not exhibit a dominant lethal effect | Hoechst (1974) |
| | male NMRI mice | 300 mg/kg gavage per day, 5 days | | did not exhibit a dominant lethal effect | Hoechst (1974) |

[a] Phenazin concentration in carbendazim: 9 ppm DAP, 5 ppm AHP

[b] Phenazin concentration in carbendazim: < 0.6 ppm DAP, < 4 ppm AHP

DAP = diaminophenazine; AHP = aminohydroxyphenazine; i.p. = intraperitoneal; NR = not reported

66 weeks for the males because of increased mortality (62 surviving controls, 32 surviving at 7500 mg/kg); females, however, received 7500 mg/kg throughout the study period. Animals were 6-7 weeks old at the start of this study. Mortality was compound-related in male mice. The high-dose males were sacrificed at week 73 because of a significant increase in mortality (23 surviving). Only nine males in the 1500-mg/kg group survived to week 104, compared with 18 surviving control males. Females did not show this increase in mortality.

There were no dose-related effects on body weight or food consumption at any time during the study, although terminal body weights for the low- and mid-dose males were less than those of the control and high-dose males. Clinical data were similar for all treatment and control groups. Haematological measures were unaffected.

Both absolute and relative thymus weights were significantly decreased in females at 500 and 1500 mg/kg, but not in the high-dose group. Absolute liver weight was increased in the high-dose females and relative liver weight at the two highest-dose levels. The organ weights of male mice were variable and only the kidney and thymus weights appeared to be decreased as a result of treatment. Absolute kidney and thymus weights were depressed in male mice at all treatment levels, but relative kidney and thymus weights were significantly decreased only in the high-dose males. Histological examination revealed dose-related changes in the thymus (lymphoid depletion) and accumulation of yellow-brown pigment in the renal tubules for mid- and high-dose male mice.

Examination of the testes demonstrated an increase in the frequency of sperm stasis in mid- and high-dose males, together with increased germinal cell atrophy (bilateral only). There was no trend, however, towards unilateral germinal cell atrophy, the incidence in controls being greater than or equal to that of treated males. These effects are, therefore, not considered to be compound-related.

The examination of male mice livers revealed a significant hepatotoxic effect at 1500 and 7500 mg/kg, demonstrated by centrilobular hypertrophy, necrosis and swelling. There was no increase in the frequency of hepatocellular adenomas; these occurred with equal frequency in control and treatment groups. There was a significant increase in hepatocellular carcinomas but only at 1500 mg/kg. However, too few males survived at the high-dose level to 17 months (510 days) to support the conclusion of no oncogenic effect at that dose level.

The occurrence of total hepatic tumours (hepatocellular carcinomas, hepatocellular adenomas and hepatoblastomas) is given in Table 10. This was statistically increased ($P < 0.05$) for the low-, mid-, and high-dose females. It was also statistically increased ($P < 0.05$) in mid-dose males but was not evaluated in high-dose males because of the high rate of mortality.

In conclusion, this study on CD-1 mice showed that there were statistically significant increases ($P < 0.05$) in the incidence of hepatocellular carcinoma at 1500 mg/kg for males and at all dose levels for females, the response being dose-related ($P < 0.05$). Because of high mortality in the high-dose males, a dose-response relationship could not be determined. In addition, the high mortality rate in male controls further hampered the interpretation of results. Histopathological analysis of the hepatocellular tumours in the test animals showed no difference from controls, and the median latent period for development of these hepatocellular carcinomas showed no significant decrease in the test animals. No carcinogenic effect was observed in tissues other than the liver (Wood, 1982).

In a study on SPF Swiss mice (100 males and 100 females per group), carbendazim was administered in the diet at dosage levels of 0, 150, 300 and 1000 mg/kg diet for 80 weeks. The highest-dose was increased to 2000 mg/kg at week 4 and to 5000 mg/kg at week 8 for the remainder of the study. Animals were examined for behaviour and clinical signs of toxicity, and body weight measurements were determined throughout the study. Gross pathology investigations were performed on all animals, liver and kidney weights were recorded, and tissues were examined microscopically. There were no compound-related effects on general condition, mortality or body weight. Survival at term was 70% for males and 80% for females. Relative liver weights for high-dose males and females were significantly different from those of controls, but there were no changes in kidney weights. The results are shown in Table 11. The combined incidence of hepatocellular adenomas and hepatocellular carcinomas increased with increasing dose levels for both males and females. Males showed a more pronounced induction of liver tumours and a more frequent occurrence of hepatocellular carcinomas which were often found simultaneously with hepatocellular adenomas. Females, on the contrary, showed only hepatocellular adenomas in most cases (Beems et al., 1976; Mohr, 1977).

Table 10. Incidence of combined primary hepatocellular tumours and mean and median period for development after treatment with carbendazim in CD-1 mice[a]

| | Male mice | | | | Female mice | | | |
|---|---|---|---|---|---|---|---|---|
| Carbendazim concentration (mg/kg diet): | 0 | 500 | 1500 | 7500 (3750) | 0 | 500 | 1500 | 7500 |
| Combined incidences of hepatic tumours | 13 | 20 | 23[b] | NA[c] | 1 | 9[b] | 21[b] | 15[b] |
| Median period for development (days) | 633 | 697 | 651 | NA[c] | 732 | 724 | 697 | 733 |
| Mean period for development (days) | 628 | 671 | 628 | NA[c] | 732 | 706 | 689 | 653 |
| Number of mice examined[d] | 80 | 80 | 80 | 80 | 79 | 78 | 80 | 78 |
| Median survival time (weeks) | 79 | 72 | 69 | 64 | 91 | 91 | 91 | 91 |
| Number of mice alive at termination | 18 | 14 | 9 | 23 | 22 | 15 | 13 | 20 |

[a] From: Wood (1982)
[b] Significant by Fisher's Exact Test at $P \leq 0.05$ level of probability
[c] NA = not applicable. This group was terminated after 516 days on test (test week 73) due to a high rate of mortality. In view of the early termination of this test group and low incidence of hepatic tumours observed in this group, the inclusion of its data in statistical evaluation of hepatic tumour incidence is considered inappropriate.
[d] Mice found dead or sacrificed *in extremis* prior to each group's termination were subjected to gross pathological evaluation.

Table 11. Incidence of proliferation lesions of the hepatocytes in Swiss mice[a]

| | Male mice | | | | Female mice | | | |
|---|---|---|---|---|---|---|---|---|
| Carbendazim concentration (mg/kg diet): | 0 | 150 | 300 | 5000 | 0 | 150 | 300 | 5000 |
| Number of animals examined[b] | 100 | 94 | 98 | 100 | 94 | 99 | 98 | 95 |
| Liver nodular hyperplasia[c] | 0 | 8 | 11 | 25 | 0 | 5 | 3 | 11 |
| Hepatocellular adenoma | 9 | 5 | 13 | 14 | 1 | 1 | 3 | 8 |
| Hepatocellular carcinoma | 1 | 3 | 4 | 9 | 1 | 0 | 0 | 0 |

[a] Adapted from: Mohr (1977)
[b] A number of animals could not be examined because of well-advanced autolysis. In addition, slides were not available for some of the animals.
[c] Values for this non-neoplastic lesion included all types of cellular alteration. A statistical analysis was not conducted.

In a study on HOE NMRKf (SPF 71) mice (100-120 males and females per group), carbendazim was administered in the diet for 96 weeks at dosage levels of 0, 50, 150, 300 and 1000 mg/kg diet. The highest-dose was increased to 2000 mg/kg at week 4 and to 5000 mg/kg at week 8 for the remainder of the study. Animals were examined for behaviour and general condition, as well as for body weight, food/water consumption and mortality. Gross necropsies were performed on all animals, liver and lung weights were recorded, and all organs and tissues were examined microscopically. An interim sacrifice was made at 18 months of 20 males and 20 females from the control group and the highest-dose group.

There were no compound-related effects on behaviour, body weight gain, food/water consumption or mortality. At 22 months there was 24-31% mortality in male mice and 37-52% mortality in females in all groups of mice. As there was no difference between the treated and control groups, it was concluded mortality was not influenced by the feeding of carbendazim. The mean daily consumption of carbendazim in mg/kg body weight for males and females, respectively, was 5.8 and 7.1 at 50 mg/kg diet, 17.1 and 21.2 at 150 mg/kg diet, 34.4 and 41.9 at 300 mg/kg diet, and 548.4 and 682.3 at 5000 mg/kg diet.

Examination of lung and liver weights at 18 and 22 months demonstrated an increase in absolute and relative liver weights in both male and female mice at 5000 mg/kg diet. Macroscopic and microscopic examination of 20 male and 20 female animals killed after 18 months of receiving 5000 mg carbendazim/kg revealed compound-related effects on the liver. All animals demonstrated centrilobular hypertrophy, single cell necrosis, mitotic cells and pigmented Kupffer cells. The tissues of the remaining 100 males and 100 females exposed to 5000 mg/kg were evaluated at 22 months. There was marked liver cell hypertrophy (greater than in animals treated for 18 months only), clear cell foci, mitosis, inclusion bodies in enlarged cell nuclei, multiple cell necrosis, and greenish yellow pigment in Kupffer cells.

Neoplastic nodules (adenomas), carcinomas, fibrosarcomas and other tumorigenic responses in the liver were equally distributed among all groups (Tables 12 and 13). Although haemangiomas of the liver (Table 14) were found in all treated groups (but not in controls), no dose-related response was evident. Lung adenomatosis was equally distributed among all groups. There was no effect of carbendazim on the incidence or time of onset of

Table 12. Incidence of tumours in HOE NMRKf mice after 18 months of exposure[a]

| | Control | | Mice treated with 5000 mg/kg diet | |
|---|---|---|---|---|
| | male | female | male | female |
| Lung | | | | |
| adenoma | 3 | 5 | 4 | - |
| Uterus | | | | |
| stromal sarcoma | | 1 | | - |
| Ovary | | | | |
| tubular adenoma | | 1 | | - |
| granulosa cell tumour | | 1 | | - |
| luteoma and tubular adenoma | | 1 | | - |
| Skin and subcutaneous tissue | | | | |
| round cell sarcoma | - | - | - | 1 |
| adenocarcinoma | - | - | 1 | - |
| Lymph nodes | | | | |
| lymphosarcoma | - | - | - | 1 |
| | 3 | 9 | 5 | 2 |

[a] Adapted from Donaubauer et al. (1982)

tumours, and the total number of benign and malignant tumours was comparable among the various groups of mice. Thus, there was no evidence of a carcinogenic effect from carbendazim when administered in the diet to mice at doses up to and including 5000 mg/kg diet for 22 months (Donaubauer et al., 1982).

## 7.8 Neurotoxicity

Carbendazim (500, 2500 and 5000 mg/kg) has been evaluated for neurotoxic potential in white Leghorn hens (10 per group). Controls consisted of the vehicle (corn oil) and the neurotoxin tri-*o*-tolyl phosphate (TOTP). The hens were observed daily for mortality and clinical neurotoxicity for four weeks. Neurotoxic signs, consisting of leg weakness, ataxia and/or "goose-stepping" gait, were observed in hens treated with TOTP. Less severe and reversible signs, consisting of slight leg weakness and ataxia, were

Table 13. Possible preneoplastic changes and primary neoplasms in the livers and lungs of HOE NMRKf mice after 22 months of exposure[a]

| Carbendazim concentration: | 0 | | 50 | | 150 | | 300 | | 5000 | |
|---|---|---|---|---|---|---|---|---|---|---|
| (mg/kg diet) | male | female | male | female | male | female | male | female | male | female |
| **Liver** | | | | | | | | | | |
| Neoplastic nodules (adenomas) | 3 | | 2 | | | | | 1 | 1 | |
| Clear cell foci | | | | | | | | | 3 | 4 |
| Basophilic foci | | | | 1 | 1 | | | | | |
| Haemangiomas (liver) | | | 2 | | 3 | | 2 | 2 | | 1 |
| **Lungs** | | | | | | | | | | |
| Adenomatosis | 29 | 10 | 31 | 8 | 30 | 10 | 25 | 9 | 22 | 12 |
| Adenocarcinomas | | | | 1 | | | | | 1 | |
| Keratinizing squamous cell carcinomas | | | | | | 1 | | | | |
| Cavernous haemangioma | | | | 1 | | | | | | |
| | 32 | 10 | 35 | 11 | 34 | 11 | 27 | 12 | 27 | 17 |

[a] Adapted from Donaubauer et al. (1982)

Table 14. Haemangiomas of the liver in HOE NMRKf mice after 22 months of exposure[a]

| Dose (mg/kg diet) | Male | Female |
|---|---|---|
| 0 | 0 | 0 |
| 50 | 2 | 0 |
| 150 | 3 | 0 |
| 300 | 2 | 2 |
| 5000 | 0 | 1 |

[a] Adapted from Donaubauer et al. (1982)

observed in hens treated with 5000 mg carbendazim/kg, but no neurotoxic signs were observed for those treated with 500 or 2500 mg/kg. Microscopic examination indicated that there was no axonal degeneration or demyelination in carbendazim-treated animals (Goldenthal, 1978).

## 7.9 Toxicity of contaminants

When manufactured under certain conditions, carbendazim contains a class of contaminants called phenazines. These contaminants are mutagenic at very low concentrations in the *Salmonella typhimurium* Ames test and also in the mouse lymphoma Y5178Y TK$^{+/-}$ gene mutation assay. Concentrations of > 4 ppm diaminophenazine or 10 ppm aminohydroxyphenazine yielded positive results. Process changes by some of carbendazim manufacturers have now removed the phenazines.

## 7.10 Mechanisms of toxicity - mode of action

Biochemical studies on the mechanism of action of benzimidazole compounds have shown that their biological effects are caused by interactions with cell microtubules (Davidse & Flach, 1977). These cellular structures are present in all eukaryotic cells and are involved in several vital functions, such as intracellular transports and cell division. Benzimidazole compounds have been used as anticancer drugs and as anthelminthic drugs in animals and humans because they act as spindle poisons by interfering with the formation and/or functioning of microtubules. However, eukaryotes are known to be unequally sensitive to each benzimidazol compound, which explains the use of these compounds in helminthiases. Selective toxicity of benomyl and carbendazim for fungi has been explained by comparing their binding to fungal and mammalian tubulin. The different sensitivity of several fungi has also been explained by the different affinity of benomyl and carbendazim for fungal tubulin.

Benomyl has been found to bind to fungal tubulin but not to porcine brain tubulin, indicating that mammalian tubulin has no, or at least low, affinity for benomyl (Davidse & Flach, 1977). This is in agreement with the observation that benomyl at concentrations that are lethal for sensitive fungi does not interact with *in vitro* microtubule assembly in these brain extracts. *In vitro* $ID_{50}$ values for several mycelial extracts of various fungal species sensitive to benomyl were all below 5 $\mu$mol/litre (Davidse & Flach, 1977). *In vitro* rat brain tubulin polymerization was inhibited to about 20% at benomyl or carbendazim concentrations of 25 $\mu$mol/litre (De Brabander et al., 1976b). For comparison, a standard antitubulin drug in humans such as vincristine inhibited 50% tubulin assembly at 0.1 $\mu$mol/litre in the same experiment. The assembly of sheep and calf brain microtubule was also found to be unaffected by carbendazim concentrations higher than 100 $\mu$mol/litre (Ireland et al., 1979).

Mitotic arrest by benzimidazole and six analogues at metaphase was evaluated in human lymphocyte cultures. Structure-activity relationships indicate that antimitotic activity is related to C6 substitution of the benzimidazole moiety (Holden et al., 1980). In this study, however, benomyl and carbendazim were not tested. The question of whether all C6 unsubstituted benzimidazoles, such as benomyl and carbendazim, have no effect on mitosis of human lymphocytes in cell cultures is therefore unresolved.

A link between the effects of benomyl and carbendazim on tubulin and their teratogenic effects has been postulated (Ellis et al., 1987, 1988).

# 8. EFFECTS ON HUMANS

## 8.1 General population exposure

No references to carbendazim poisoning have been documented in the literature. Recent data to estimate dietary exposure of the benzimidazole benomyl, based on food consumption patterns within the USA and elsewhere, indicate exposure below the NOELs from animal toxicity tests. Further information is given in section 5.2.1 of Environmental Health Criteria 148: Benomyl (WHO, 1993).

## 8.2 Occupational exposure

Selected blood profiles from 50 factory workers involved in the manufacture of benomyl and carbendazim were compared to those of a control group of 48 workers who were not exposed to these two fungicides. White blood cell count, red blood cell count, and haemoglobin and haematocrit values were comparable among the two groups. There were no quantitative estimates of exposure given for the factory workers. No female employees were included in the control group (Everhart, 1979; FAO/WHO, 1985a).

A study was performed to determine whether exposure to benomyl and carbendazim had an adverse effect on the fertility of 298 male manufacturing workers exposed to benomyl between 1970 and 1977. The workers ranged from 19 to 64 years of age (79% were between 20 and 39, and 78% of the spouses were similarly aged between 20 and 39 years). Exposure duration ranged from less than one month to 95 months, and more than 51% of the workers were potentially exposed from 1 to 5 months. The birth rates of exposed workers' spouses were compared with those of four comparison populations from the same county, state, region and country (USA). There was no reduction in fertility as shown by the birth rates for the study population, which were generally higher than the comparison populations. Spermatogenesis among workers was not examined (Gooch, 1978; FAO/WHO, 1985a).

# 9. EFFECTS ON OTHER ORGANISMS IN THE LABORATORY AND FIELD

## 9.1 Microorganisms

Studies on soil effects have concentrated on benomyl. However, carbendazim, the breakdown product of benomyl, would be expected to produce comparable results.

Soil respiration has been found to be little influenced by benomyl at concentrations below 10 mg/kg, which is the maximum soil concentration expected after use at recommended application rates (Hofer et al., 1971; van Fassen, 1974; Peeples, 1974; Weeks & Hedrick, 1975).

A study on the influence of benomyl on soil nitrogen mineralization showed that the release of ammonia was not decreased by benomyl, whereas the influence of the fungicide on nitrification varied from a stimulation (van Fassen, 1974), through no effect (Mazur & Hughes, 1975), to a decreased nitrification (Hofer et al., 1971; Wainwright & Pugh, 1974). The differences may be related to the soil composition since Hofer et al. (1971) found a greater effect in sandy than in organic soil.

Benomyl, in combination with eleven other pesticides that were used in an orchard spray programme, had only a minimal and short-term effect on respiration, ammonification and nitrification at concentrations expected after recommended use of benomyl over a spraying season. Ten times the recommended application rates had a pronounced effect on both respiration and nitrification, which lasted for more than 4 weeks (Helweg, 1985).

The influence of benomyl and carbendazim on soil microbial activity was studied in Sweden following repeated annual applications during autumn to winter cereals for a period of 3 to 5 years. The effects of the fungicides on straw decomposition, balance of straw fungal flora and nitrogen mineralization in the soil were investigated in field and laboratory experiments. The decomposition of straw in the field was not affected in clay soils by annual applications of up to 2 kg/ha. In sandy soils, rates of up to 0.5 kg/ha had no effect, but in one case at 2 kg/ha the initial stages of straw decomposition were slightly inhibited. All doses tested in both clay and sandy soils caused changes in the composition of the straw fungal flora (Torstensson & Wessen, 1984).

Tests were conducted to determine the effects of the fungicide carbendazim (Bavistin), the herbicide fluometuron (Cotoran) and the insecticide curacron on Egyptian soil fungi when applied at the recommended field rates and at 4 and 8 times these rates. Carbendazim produced a significant inhibition of the total count of fungi at all three rates after 5 and 40 days and at the higher application rates after 80 days. The response of *Aspergillus* sp. alone to this fungicide reflected the effects on the total fungal count (Abdel-Fattah et al., 1982).

An application of carbendazim (5 mg formulation/kg soil) and Calixin (1.5 mg formulation/kg soil) significantly enhanced the microbial activity, as well as the availability of ammonium nitrogen and phosphate in the soil, while nitrite, nitrate and available potassium were found to decrease. During incubation, $CO_2$ evolution decreased during the first 21 days, increased up to 42 days, and, thereafter, decreased with both treatments (Khan et al., 1987).

## 9.2 Aquatic organisms

The effect of carbendazim was monitored using the green alga *Selenastrum capricornutum* in an OECD guideline test (201). The $EC_{50}$ (based on total growth) at 72 h was 1.3 mg/litre and at 120 h was 1.6 mg/litre. The no-observed-effect concentration (NOEC) was 0.5 mg/litre. To study whether carbendazim was algistatic or algicidal, organisms were recultured at the end of the initial 120 h of incubation. Regrowth occurred in the control but not in the test cultures (8.0 mg/litre) after a period of 9 days. Carbendazim was, therefore, considered to be algicidal (Douglas & Handley, 1987). In another study using *Chlorella pyrenoidosa*, the 48-h $EC_{50}$ for growth inhibition was calculated to be 0.54 mg/litre (Canton, 1976).

The acute toxicity of carbendazim to a variety of aquatic organisms is summarized in Table 15. For 96-h tests, $LC_{50}$ values ranged from 0.007 mg/litre for channel catfish (*Ictalurus punctatus* yolk-sac fry) to 5.5 mg/litre for bluegill sunfish (Palawski & Knowles, 1986).

In a static renewal 21-day test using *Daphnia magna*, onset of reproduction was the most sensitive indicator, being significantly delayed at 0.025 mg carbendazim/litre (measured concentration). Other parameters (number of days reproducing, total number of young, and young produced per day) were affected significantly at 0.05 mg/litre. The NOEC was 0.013 mg/litre (measured concentration) (Hutton et al., 1986).

Gillet & Roubaud (1983) showed that the toxicity of carbendazim to carp (*Cyprinus carpio*) was greater for the fertilization and early development stages than for the adult stages. They found the 30-min $LC_{100}$ during the fertilization stage to be < 5 mg/litre at pH 9 and < 2.5 mg/litre at pH 7. The rainbow trout (*Oncorhynchus mykiss*) was more sensitive, with an $LC_{100}$ (30 min, pH 9) of 0.5 mg/litre and 71% survival, compared to controls, at 0.05 mg/litre.

Bluegill sunfish were exposed to benomyl, carbendazim and 2-AB at concentrations of 0.05 mg/litre (measured concentrations 0.01 to 0.04 mg/litre) and 5.0 mg/litre (measured concentration 2 to 5 mg/litre). No residue was found in the tissues of fish exposed to low levels of these compounds, but detectable residues were found in the tissues of fish exposed to the high levels. However, there was no build-up or bioconcentration with time (DuPont, 1972).

## 9.3 Terrestrial organisms

Van Gestel et al. (1992) exposed red earthworms (*Eisenia andrei*) to carbendazim, added as an aqueous solution of the formulation Derosal, to artificial soil. The final concentrations in soil were 0, 1, 3.2, 10, 32 and 100 mg formulation/kg dry soil, corresponding to 0, 0.6, 1.92, 6.0, 19.2 and 60 mg carbendazim/kg. The worms had been acclimatised for 1 week in the artificial soil, which contained 8 g cow dung per kg soil as food for the worms. The soil pH (7.3) was higher than optimum for this species and resulted in a lower cocoon production in this test than expected. At the two highest concentrations of 19.2 and 60 mg a.i./kg, all worms died over the 3 week experimental period; an $LC_{50}$ of 5.7 (4.7-6.9) mg a.i./kg was calculated. Growth was significantly reduced at 6.0 mg/kg soil, and reproduction (measured as cocoon production, number of fertile cocoons and numbers of juveniles) was significantly reduced at ≥ 1.92 mg a.i./kg soil. The $EC_{50}$ for cocoon production was calculated to be 2.9 (2.2-3.8) mg a.i./kg dry soil. The response curve for reproduction and growth effects of carbendazim was steep. Vonk et al. (1986) had reported comparable results for a second *Eisenia* species, *E. foetida*, in a different artifical soil; the $LC_{50}$ was 9.3 mg/kg soil and the NOEC for cocoon production 2.0 mg/kg soil.

Table 15. Toxicity of carbendazim to aquatic organisms

| Organism | Size/[a] age | Stat/ flow | Temperature (°C) | Hardness[b] (mg/litre) | pH | Duration (h) | $LC_{50}$ (mg/litre) | Reference |
|---|---|---|---|---|---|---|---|---|
| **Freshwater** | | | | | | | | |
| Water flea | < 24 h | stat | 20 | 179 | 7.5 | 48 | 0.087 | Hutton (1988) |
| *(Daphnia magna)* | < 24 h | stat | 20 | | | 48 | 0.46 | Canton (1976) |
| Rainbow trout | 3 months | stat | 15 | | | 48 | 1.8 | Canton (1976) |
| *(Oncorhynchus mykiss)* | 0.8 g | stat | 13 | | 7.5 | 96 | 0.36 | Heinemann (1971) |
| | yolk-sac fry | stat | 10 | 40-48 | 7.4 | 96 | 0.145 | Palawski & Knowles (1986) |
| | swimup fry | stat | 10 | 40-48 | 7.4 | 96 | 0.32 | Palawski & Knowles (1986) |
| | 0.2 g | stat | 10 | 40-48 | 7.4 | 96 | 0.37 | Palawski & Knowles (1986) |
| | 1.2 g | stat | 10 | 40-48 | 7.4 | 96 | 0.87 | Palawski & Knowles (1986) |
| | | stat | 12 | 40-48 | 7.4 | 96 | > 1.8 | Palawski & Knowles (1986) |
| | | stat | 17 | 40-48 | 7.4 | 96 | 0.87 | Palawski & Knowles (1986) |
| | | stat | 22 | 40-48 | 7.4 | 96 | 0.1 | Palawski & Knowles (1986) |
| | | stat | 10 | 40-48 | 6.5 | 96 | 0.64 | Palawski & Knowles (1986) |
| | | stat | 10 | 40-48 | 7.5 | 96 | 0.41 | Palawski & Knowles (1986) |
| | | stat | 10 | 40-48 | 8.5 | 96 | 0.34 | Palawski & Knowles (1986) |
| | | stat | 10 | 40 | 7.4 | 96 | 0.78 | Palawski & Knowles (1986) |
| | | stat | 10 | 320 | 7.4 | 96 | 0.88 | Palawski & Knowles (1986) |

Table 15 (contd).

| | | | | | | | | |
|---|---|---|---|---|---|---|---|---|
| Bluegill sunfish | 0.95 g | stat | 22-23 | 67 | 7.0 | 96 | 5.5 | Wetzel & Hutton (1984) |
| *(Lepomis macrochirus)* | 0.2 g | stat | 22 | 40-48 | 7.4 | 96 | > 3.2 | Palawski & Knowles (1986) |
| Channel catfish | yolk-sac fry | stat | 22 | 40-48 | 7.4 | 96 | 0.007 | Palawski & Knowles (1986) |
| *(Ictalurus punctatus)* | swimup fry | stat | 22 | 40-48 | 7.4 | 96 | 0.012 | Palawski & Knowles (1986) |
| | 0.2 g | stat | 22 | 40-48 | 7.4 | 96 | 0.01 | Palawski & Knowles (1986) |
| | 1.2 g | stat | 22 | 40-48 | 7.4 | 96 | 0.019 | Palawski & Knowles (1986) |
| | | stat | 12 | 40-48 | 7.4 | 96 | > 0.56 | Palawski & Knowles (1986) |
| | | stat | 17 | 40-48 | 7.4 | 96 | 0.14 | Palawski & Knowles (1986) |
| | | stat | 22 | 40-48 | 7.4 | 96 | 0.032 | Palawski & Knowles (1986) |
| | | stat | 22 | 40-48 | 6.5 | 96 | 0.023 | Palawski & Knowles (1986) |
| | | stat | 22 | 40-48 | 7.5 | 96 | 0.014 | Palawski & Knowles (1986) |
| | | stat | 22 | 40-48 | 8.5 | 96 | 0.023 | Palawski & Knowles (1986) |
| | | stat | 22 | 40 | 7.4 | 96 | 0.018 | Palawski & Knowles (1986) |
| | | stat | 22 | 320 | 7.4 | 96 | 0.024 | Palawski & Knowles (1986) |
| Toad | tadpole | stat | 25 | | | 48 | 3.5 | Nishiuchi & Yoshida (1974) |
| *(Bufo bufo japonicus)* | | | | | | | | |

Table 15 (contd).

| Organism | Size/[a] age | Stat/ flow | Tempera- ture (°C) | Hardness[b] (mg/litre) | pH | Duration (h) | $LC_{50}$ (mg/litre) | Reference |
|---|---|---|---|---|---|---|---|---|
| **Marine and Estuarine** | | | | | | | | |
| Eastern oyster (*Crassostrea virginica*) | 25-50 mm | flow | 18-20 | | | 96 | > 1.145[c] | Boeri (1988a) |
| Mysid shrimp (*Mysidopsis bahia*) | | stat | 23 | | | 96 | 0.098 | Boeri (1988c) |
| Sheepshead minnow (*Cyprinodon variegatus*) | 0.14 g | stat | 22 | | | 96 | > 1.158 | Boeri (1988b) |

[a] stat = static conditons (water unchanged for duration of test); flow = flow-through conditions (carbendazim concentration in water continuously maintained)
[b] hardness given as mg $CaCO_3$/litre
[c] $EC_{50}$ based on rate of shell deposition

Carbendazim (99.3% purity) was evaluated for acute contact toxicity after thoracic application in honey-bees (*Apis mellifera*). Each treatment level consisted of four replicates of ten bees each. Forty bees served as positive control (using carbaryl) and forty as negative control. No deaths occurred after the application of 50 μg carbendazim/bee, the highest rate tested. Carbendazim is, therefore, classified as "relatively non-toxic" to the honey-bee (Meade, 1984).

The $LD_{50}$ for bobwhite quail, with an observation period of 14 days following the single oral dose, was > 2250 mg/kg body weight (Beavers, 1985). For mallard ducks the dietary 5-day $LC_{50}$ was > 10 000 mg carbendazim/kg diet (Fink, 1975).

## 9.4 Population and ecosystem effects

Van Gestel (1992) has summarized reports of toxicity of carbendazim on earthworms from field studies based on different soil types, application rates and crops (Table 16). Estimated soil concentrations in this table are based on application rates; it has been assumed that there is no mobility of the compound beyond the top 2.5 cm of soil and homogeneous distribution of carbendazim in this layer. For orchard application, it was further assumed that 50% of the applied active ingredient reached the soil. Reported effects include reduced numbers, reduced activity (as reduced removal of leaf litter) and reduced reproduction of worms. Application rates were within the recommended rates for carbendazim as a fungicide on these crops.

Table 16. Summary of earthworm toxicity data on carbendazim in field studies

| Crop/soil type | Dosage (kg/ha) | Estimated soil concentration (mg/kg) | Time (days) | Effect | Reference |
|---|---|---|---|---|---|
| Grass | 0.3 | 0.9 | 12 | 11% reduction in number | Ammon (1985) |
| Grass | 0.56 | 1.6 | 49 | 72% reduction in cast production<br>42% more litter left | Keogh & Whitehead (1975) |
| Winter wheat/clay | 0.15 | 0.4 | 275 | 14% reduction in juveniles<br>50% increase in adult *Allolobophora caliginosa* | Lofs-Holmin (1981) |
| | | | | 25% increase in juveniles<br>25% reduction in adult *A. chlorotica* | Lofs-Holmin (1981) |
| Apples/loam | 0.375[a] | 1.6 | 245 | reduction in litter removal | Cook & Swait (1975) |

[a] Three separate applications of carbendazim

# 10. EVALUATION OF HUMAN HEALTH RISKS AND EFFECTS ON THE ENVIRONMENT

Benomyl and carbendazim are two different fungicides in their own right. However, carbendazim is also the main metabolite of benomyl in mammals and the degradation product of benomyl in the environment. Butyl isocyanate is the chemical moiety removed from benomyl when carbendazim is formed. Given the similar toxicities caused by benomyl and carbendazim and the different toxicological profile of butyl isocyanate, the two fungicides are evaluated together in this monograph.

## 10.1 Evaluation of human health risks

The two primary routes of exposure to humans are through diet and through manufacturing or use of the product.

There is limited information on actual dietary exposure to benomyl and carbendazim. Dietary exposure has been estimated in the Netherlands and the USA. In the USA, exposure based on dietary habits, measured residue levels, and the percentage of crop treated has been calculated for various subgroups of population. These calculations indicate that the estimated benomyl exposure is 0.144-1.479 μg/kg per day (section 5.2.1 of Environmental Health Criteria 148: Benomyl (WHO, 1993)). In the Netherlands, the mean dietary intake was estimated to be 0.83 μg/kg per day (0.05 mg/day per person). These levels of exposure are below the recommended ADI of 0.01 (carbendazim) and 0.02 (benomyl) mg/kg body weight.

The average air levels of benomyl and carbendazim have been determined in a manufacturing facility (section 5.3) and found to be less than 0.2 and 0.3 $mg/m^3$, respectively. Both values are below the Threshold Limit Value of 5-10 mg $benomyl/m^3$ established by a number of governmental agencies.

In one study, potential respiratory and dermal exposure to benomyl wettable powder formulation was determined under several agricultural use situations (section 5.3). The highest rates of exposure occurred in situations of mixing and loading in preparation for aerial application; dermal and respiratory exposures were, respectively, 26 and 0.08 mg/person per cycle. Home users and agricultural workers re-entering treated fields were estimated to be exposed to about 1 mg/person per cycle and 5.9 mg/person per hour, principally through the dermal route.

Because of the low mammalian toxicity, acute benomyl or carbendazim poisonings are unlikely to occur under conditions of normal use.

Several studies of agricultural workers (section 8.2 of Environmental Health Criteria 148: Benomyl (WHO, 1993)) have shown some cases of contact dermatitis after exposure to benomyl. These effects can be significantly reduced or eliminated by wearing long-sleeved shirts, long trousers and gloves.

There is little information on health effects in humans as a consequence of exposure to either benomyl or carbendazim. Two studies have been conducted on factory workers involved in the manufacture of benomyl (section 8.2). In one study, haematological profiles from 50 factory workers involved in the manufacture of benomyl were comparable to those from a control group of 48 workers. A second study found no decrease in the birth rate of the wives of 298 factory workers exposed to benomyl.

Extensive studies of various species of laboratory animals show reproductive, developmental, mutagenic and carcinogenic effects associated with both benomyl and carbendazim. The effects observed on rat fetuses were microphthalmia, hydrocephaly and encephaloceles. The no-observed-effect levels (NOEL) of benomyl for developmental toxicity are equal to or greater than 10 mg/kg body weight per day, depending upon the species and route of administration. Similarly, the NOEL of benomyl for reproductive effects in the male rat appears to be 15 mg/kg body weight per day after gavage dosing. In feeding studies with both benomyl and carbendazim, the NOEL appears to be 500 mg/kg diet (equivalent to 25 mg/kg body weight per day). However, one benomyl feeding study reported a NOEL of less than 1 mg/kg diet (0.05 mg/kg body weight per day) for male reproductive effects. The reason for the discrepancy between the NOEL in this latter study and other investigations is unknown.

The only consistent genotoxic effect noted in animal studies is the induction of numerical chromosomal aberrations. These effects are consistent with the interaction of benomyl and carbendazim with microtubule formation.

Rat carcinogenicity studies did not show any carcinogenic effect for either compound. Benomyl and carbendazim induce hepatocellular tumours in CD-1 and SPF Swiss mice but not in NMRKf mice. This finding in mice is not considered to be a result of a direct genotoxic action. Rather, it appears to be associated with liver toxicity in strains of mice that are highly susceptible to tumour formation at this site.

Benomyl and carbendazim are spindle poisons. Effects on target cells are consequences of binding to microtubules, giving toxicities similar to those of other spindle poisons such as colchicine and vincristine. Benzimidazole compounds in general and benomyl and carbendazim in particular have selective effects on the microtubules of different eukaryotes. Reasons for this selectivity include the binding capability to different tubulins and pharmacokinetic differences across species. *In vitro* concentrations of benomyl used to kill sensitive fungi were found to be ineffective in disturbing mammalian microtubular functions. These studies on the mechanism of action of benomyl and carbendazim indicate a selective effect of these compounds for target species.

In summary, the $LD_{50}$, as determined in a number of test species, for benomyl ranges from > 2000 to > 12 000 mg/kg and for carbendazim from > 2000 to > 15 000 mg/kg. There are no known reports of human poisoning for either compound. This, coupled with the low estimated environmental levels of both compounds, would suggest that the possibility of acute poisoning by benomyl or carbendazim is very remote. Similarly, the data available on test species make it unlikely that either benomyl or carbendazim is carcinogenic for humans. The NOELs for both reproductive and teratogenic effects of benomyl and carbendazim (i.e. 10-15 mg/kg) do raise a possibility that an accidental ingestion of either fungicide could adversely alter reproductive outcome in humans, but the likelihood that such poisoning would occur is remote. The selectivity of these two benzimidazole compounds for the tubulin of the target species (fungi) and their relative ineffectiveness to disturb mammalian microtubule function further reduce the possibility of their having toxic effects in humans.

## 10.2 Evaluation of effects on the environment

Benomyl is rapidly converted to carbendazim in various environmental compartments, the half-lives being 2 and 19 h in water and soil, respectively. Therefore, data from studies on both benomyl and carbendazim are relevant for the evaluation of environmental effects.

Carbendazim persists on leaf surfaces and in leaf litter. In soil the half-life is between 3 and 12 months, and the compound may be detected for up to 3 years. However, in many cases, major residues will be lost within a single season. Residues of carbendazim and its metabolites are strongly bound or incorporated into soil organic matter. The strong adsorption ($K_{oc}$ = approximately 2000) of carbendazim to soil and sediment particles reduces its bioavailability to terrestrial and aquatic organisms. Similarly, the mobility of carbendazim in soil is limited, and it is not expected to leach to ground water.

Benomyl and carbendazim are highly toxic to some aquatic organisms in laboratory tests, the most sensitive species being the channel catfish with a 96-h $LC_{50}$ for yolk-sac fry of 0.006 mg benomyl/litre. However, this toxicity is unlikely to be manifest in the environment for most aquatic organisms because of the low bioavailability in surface waters. The exposure of sediment-living organisms could be greater, but no test results are available for these organisms.

Benomyl and carbendazim affect groups of fungi in soil but do not seem to modify the overall microbial activity of the soil when used at normal field rates.

In both the laboratory and field, benomyl and carbendazim applied at recommended rates cause deaths and sublethal reproductive effects on earthworms of many different species. Surface-feeding species eating leaf litter are most at risk. Populations may take more than 2 years to recover. There are no studies available on other litter and soil invertebrates.

Benomyl and carbendazim have low toxicity for birds and carbendazim is classified as "relatively non-toxic" to honey-bees.

## 10.3 Conclusions

Benomyl causes dermal sensitization in humans. Both benomyl and carbendazim represent a very low risk for acute poisoning in humans. Given the current exposures and the low rate of dermal absorption of benomyl and carbendazim, it is unlikely that they would cause systemic toxicity effects either in the general population or in occupationally exposed subjects. These conclusions are drawn from animal data and from the limited human data available, but these extrapolations are supported by the understanding of the mode of action of carbendazim and benomyl in both target and non-target species.

Further elucidation of the mechanism of toxicity of carbendazim and benomyl in mammals will perhaps permit a better determination of no-observed-effect levels. Binding studies on tubulins of target cells (testis and embryonic tissues) will facilitate comparisons across species.

Carbendazim is strongly adsorbed to soil organic matter and remains in the soil for up to 3 years. It persists on leaf surfaces and, therefore, in leaf litter. Earthworms have been shown to be adversely affected (population and reproductive effects) at recommended application rates. There is no information on other soil or litter arthropods that would be similarly exposed.

The high toxicity to aquatic organisms in laboratory tests is unlikely to be seen in the field because of the low bioavailability of sediment-bound residues of carbendazim. However, no information is available on sediment-living species which would receive the highest exposure.

# 11. FURTHER RESEARCH

1. Comparative binding studies of carbendazim to tubulins of target tissues from various species should be undertaken.

2. Further clarification of the fate of 1,2-diaminobenzene and bound residues in the environment is needed.

3. The effects of benomyl and carbendazim on sediment-dwelling organisms needs to be investigated.

## 12. PREVIOUS EVALUATIONS BY INTERNATIONAL BODIES

Carbendazim was evaluated by the Joint FAO/WHO Meeting on Pesticide Residues (JMPR) in 1973, 1976, 1977, 1978, 1983 and 1988. The 1978 meeting agreed that the MRLs for benomyl, carbendazim and thiophanate-methyl should be combined and expressed as carbendazim. Carbendazim residues were last evaluated by the 1988 meeting (FAO/WHO, 1988b) and the MRLs were updated at that time. These MRLs (expressed as carbendazim) are listed in Table 4. The 1983 meeting (FAO/WHO, 1985a) evaluated carbendazim toxicology and set the following NOEL levels and ADI:

Rat: 500 mg/kg diet, equivalent to 25 mg/kg body weight

Dog: 100 mg/kg diet, equivalent to 2.5 mg/kg body weight

Rat: teratology - 30 mg/kg body weight per day (benomyl)

The estimated ADI for carbendazim was established to be 0-0.01 mg/kg body weight.

Carbendazim has not been evaluated by the International Agency for Research on Cancer (IARC).

## REFERENCES

Abdel-Fattah HM, Abdel-Kader M, & Hamida S (1982) Effect of Bavistin, Cotoran and Curacron on Egyptian soil fungi. Mycopathologia, **80**(2): 101-106.

Albertini S (1989) Influence of different factors on the induction of chromosome malsegregation in *Saccharomyces cerevisiae* D61.M by Bavistan and assessment of its genotoxic property in the Ames test and in *Saccharomyces cerevisiae* D7. Mutat Res, **216**: 327-340.

Albertini S (1991) Reevaluation of the 9 compounds reported conclusive positive in yeast *Saccharomyces cerevisiae* aneuploidy test systems by the Gene-Tox Program using strain D61.M of *Saccharomyces cerevisiae*. Mutat Res, **260**: 165-180.

Alverez L (1987) Teratogenicity study of INE-965 (carbendazim) in rats. Newark, Delaware, E.I. Du Pont de Nemours and Co., Inc., Haskell Laboratory (Unpublished report No. HLR 281-87).

Amacher DE, Paillet S, & Ray VA (1979) Point mutations at the thymidine kinase locus in L5178Y mouse lymphoma cells: Application to genetic toxicological testing. Mutat Res, **64**: 391-406.

Ames BN, McCann J, & Yamasaki E (1975) Methods of detecting carcinogens and mutagens with the Salmonella/mammalian microsome mutagenicity test. Mutat Res, **31**: 347-364.

Ammon HU (1985) Worm toxicity tests using *Tubifex tubifex*. In: Comportement et effets secondaires des pesticides dans le sol. Les Colloques de l'INRA 31, Versailles, 4-8 juin 1984. Paris, Institut national de la Recherche agronomique, pp 303-317.

Arce GT (1984a) Mutagenicity evaluation in *Salmonella typhimurium*. Newark, Delaware, E.I. Du Pont de Nemours and Co., Inc., Haskell Laboratory (Unpublished report No. HLR 72-84).

Arce GT (1984b) Mutagenicity evaluation in *Salmonella typhimurium*. Newark, Delaware, E.I. Du Pont de Nemours and Co., Inc., Haskell Laboratory (Unpublished report No. HLR 71-84).

Arthur MF, Marsh BH, Fadel LC, & Zwick TC (1989a) Anaerobic aquatic metabolism of [phenyl(U)-$^{14}$C] benomyl in West Jefferson, Ohio, pond water and sediment (Battelle Project No. N-0799-8800). Columbus, Ohio, Battelle, Environmental Sciences Department (Unpublished report No. AMR 770-87, prepared for E.I. Du Pont de Nemours and Co., Inc.).

Arthur MF, Schweitzer KL, Fadel LC, Marsh BH, & Marsh SS (1989b) Aerobic aquatic metabolism of [phenyl(U)-$^{14}$C] benomyl in Greenville, Mississippi, water and sediment (Battelle Project No. N-0966-7301). Columbus, Ohio, Battelle, Environmental Sciences Department (Unpublished report No. AMR 1452-89, prepared for E.I. Du Pont de Nemours and Co., Inc.).

Bamburg JR, Shooter EM, & Wilson L (1973) Developmental changes in microtubule protein of the chick brain. Biochemistry, **12**: 1476-1482.

Banduhn N & Obe G (1985) Mutagenicity of methyl 2-benzimidazolecarbamate, diethylstilbestrol and estradiol: Structural chromosomal aberrations, sister-chromatid exchanges, C-mitoses, polyploidies and micronuclei. Mutat Res, **156**: 199-218.

BASF (1975) Dominant lethal study: mice. Ludwigshafen, Germany, BASF AG.

Baude FJ, Gardiner JA, & Han JC-Y (1973) Characterization of residues on plants following foliar spray applications of benomyl. J Agric Food Chem, **21**: 1084-1090.

Baude FJ, Pease HL, & Holt RF (1974) Fate of benomyl on field soil and turf. J Agric Food Chem, **22**: 413.

Beavers JB (1985) An acute oral toxicity study in the bobwhite quail with H-15,607 (MBC). St. Michaels, Maryland, Wildlife International Ltd (Unpublished report No. HLO 96-85, prepared for E.I. Du Pont de Nemours and Co., Inc.).

Beems RB, Til HP, & van der Heijden CA (1976) Carcinogenicity study with carbendazim (99% MBC) in mice. The Hague, Central Institute for Nutrition and Food Research (TNO) (Summary Report No. R-4936, prepared for Hoechst AG, Frankfurt and BASF AG, Ludwigshafen).

Boeri RL (1988a) Flow through acute toxicity of carbendazim technical to the eastern oyster, *Crassostrea virginica*. Marblehead, Massachusetts, Enseco (Unpublished report No. HLO 15-89, prepared for E.I. Du Pont de Nemours and Co., Inc.).

Boeri RL (1988b) Static acute toxicity of carbendazim technical to the sheepshead minnow, *Cyprinodon variegatus*. Marblehead, Massachusetts, Enseco (Unpublished report No. HLO 12-89, prepared for E.I. Du Pont de Nemours and Co., Inc.).

Boeri RL (1988c) Static acute toxicity of carbendazim technical to the mysid, *Mysidopsis bahia*. Marblehead, Massachusetts, Enseco (Unpublished report No. HLO 829-88, prepared for E.I. Du Pont de Nemours and Co., Inc.).

Bushway RJ, Hurst HL, Kugabalasooriar J, & Perkins LB (1991) Determination of carbendazim in blueberries by reversed-phase high performance liquid chromatography. J Chromatogr, **555**: 321-324.

Canton JH (1976) The toxicity of benomyl, thiophanate-methyl, and BLM to four freshwater organisms. Bull Environ Contam Toxicol, **16**: 214-218.

Carter SD, Hess RA, & Laskey JW (1987) The fungicide methyl 2-benzimidazolecarbamate causes infertility in male Sprague-Dawley rats. Biol Reprod, **37**(3): 709-718.

Chiba M & Veres DF (1981) Fate of benomyl and its degradation compound methyl 2-benzimidazole carbamate on apple foliage. J Agric Food Chem, **29**: 588-590.

Christian MS, Hoberman AM, & Feussner EL (1985) Developmental toxicity study of carbendazim administered via gavage to New Zealand white rabbits. Horsham, Pennsylvania, Argus Research Laboratories, Inc. (Unpublished report No. HLO 515-85, prepared for E.I. Du Pont de Nemours and Co., Inc.).

Clive D, Johnson KO, Spector JFS, Batson AG, & Moore-Brown MM (1979) Validation and characterization of the L5178Y/TK +/- mouse lymphoma mutagen assay system. Mutat Res, **59**: 61-108.

Cook ME & Swait AAJ (1975) Effects of some fungicide treatments on earthworm populations and leaf removal in apple orchards. J Hortic Sci, **50**: 495-499.

County Natwest Woodmac (1992) The fungicide market. London, County Natwest Woodmac, Agrochemical Service, pp 49-51.

Cox DM & Puck TT (1969) Chromosomal non-disjunction: The action of colcemid on Chinese hamster ovary cells *in vitro*. Cytogenetics, **8**: 158-169.

Cummings AM, Harris ST, & Rehnberg GL (1990) Effects of methyl benzimidazole carbamate during early pregnancy in the rat. Fundam Appl Toxicol, **15**: 528-535.

Cummings AM, Ebron-McCoy MT, Rogers JM, Barbee BD, & Harris ST (1992) Developmental effects of methyl benzimidazole carbamate following exposure during early pregnancy. Fundam Appl Toxicol, **18**: 288-293.

Dashiell OL (1975) Oral $LD_{50}$ test in guinea pigs (Carbendazim). Newark, Delaware, E.I. Du Pont de Nemours and Co., Inc., Haskell Laboratory (Unpublished report No. HLR 846-74).

Davidse LC (1973) Antimitotic activity of methyl benzimidazol-2-yl carbamate (MBC) in *Aspergillus nidulans*. Pestic Biochem Physiol, **3**: 317-325.

Davidse LC (1975) Antimitotic activity of methyl benzimidazol-2-ylcarbamate in fungi and its binding to cellular protein. In: Borgers M & de Brabander M ed. Microtubules and microtubule inhibitors. Amsterdam, Elsevier/North-Holland Publishing Company, pp 483-495.

Davidse LC & Flach W (1977) Differential binding of methyl benzimidazol-2-yl carbamate to fungal tubulin as a mechanism of resistance to this antimitotic agent in mutant strains of *Aspergillus nidulans*. J Cell Biol, **72**: 174-193.

Davidse LC & Flach W (1978) Interaction of thiabendazole with fungal tubulin. Biochim Biophys Acta, **543**: 82-90.

Delatour P & Besse S (1990) Benzimidazole carbamate d'éthyle: effet tératogène et présence dans le lait de vache après administration de thiophanate. Ann Rech Vét, **21**: 87-92.

Delp CJ (1980) Coping with resistance to plant disease control agents. Plant Dis, **64**: 652-657.

De Brabander M, van de Veire R, Aerts F, Geuens S, & Hoebeke J (1976a) A new culture model facilitating rapid quantitative testing of mitotic spindle inhibition in mammalian cells. J Natl Cancer Inst, **56**: 357-363.

De Brabander M, van de Veire R, Aerts F, Brogers M, & Janssen PAJ (1976b) The effect of methyl[5(2-thienylcarbonyl)-1H-benzimidazol-2-yl carbamate (R17934; NSC 238159), a new synthetic antitumoral drug interfering with microtubules, on mammalian cells cultured *in vitro*. Cancer Res, **36**: 905-916.

De Vos RH, van Dokkum W, Olthof PDA, Quirijns JK, Muys T, & van der Poll JM (1984) Pesticides and other chemical residues in Dutch total diet samples (June 1976 - July 1978). Food Chem Toxicol, **22**: 11-21.

Donaubauer HH, Schuetz E, Weigand W, & Kramer M (1982) Repeated dose (24 month) feeding study for determination of the carcinogenic effect of HOE 17411 OFAT204 (carbendazim) in mice. Frankfurt, Germany, Hoechst AG, Pharmaceuticals Research, Toxicology Section (Unpublished report).

Donovan SD (1982) Mutagenicity evaluation in *Salmonella typhimurium*. Newark, Delaware, E.I. Du Pont de Nemours and Co., Inc., Haskell Laboratory (Unpublished report No. HLR 678-82).

Donovan SM (1983) Mutagenicity evaluation in *Salmonella typhimurium*. Newark, Delaware, E.I. Du Pont de Nemours and Co., Inc., Haskell Laboratory (Unpublished report No. HLR 797-82).

Dorn E, Schmidt E, Kellner HM, & Leist KH (1983) HOE 017411-14-C (carbendazim-14-C) metabolic fate in rats and mice, a comparison. Frankfurt, Germany, Hoechst AG.

Douglas MT & Handley JW (1987) The algistatic activity of carbendazim technical. Huntingdon, United Kingdom, Huntingdon Research Centre Ltd (Unpublished report No. DPT 171(g)/871604, prepared for E.I. Du Pont de Nemours and Co., Inc.).

Du Pont (1972) Residue studies - fish: benomyl, MBC, and 2-AB. Wilmington, Delaware, E.I. Du Pont de Nemours and Co., Inc. (Unpublished report).

Eckert J, Stauffer R, & Hoppman D (1985) Determination of MBC, 4-OH MBC, and 5-OH MBC in chicken eggs, tissues and feces. Bernville, Pennsylvania, Enviro-Bio-Tech Ltd (Unpublished report No. AMR 260-84, prepared for E.I. Du Pont de Nemours and Co., Inc.).

Edwards DF (1974a) Skin absorption $LD_{50}$ (carbendazim). Newark, Delaware, Du Pont de Nemours and Co., Inc., Haskell Laboratory (Unpublished report No. HLR 798-74).

Edwards DF (1974b) Federal Hazardous Substances Act - Eye irritation test in rabbits (carbendazim). Newark, Delaware, E.I. Du Pont de Nemours and Co., Inc., Haskell Laboratory (Unpublished report No. HLR 799-74).

Ellis WG, Semple JL, Hoogenboom ER, Kavlock RJ, & Zeman FJ (1987) Benomyl-induced craniocerebral anomalies in fetuses of adequately nourished and protein-deprived rats. Teratog Carcinog Mutagen, 7: 357-375.

Ellis WG, De Roos F, Kavlock RJ, & Zeman FJ (1988) Relationship of periventricular overgrowth to hydrocephalus in brains of fetal rats exposed to benomyl. Teratog Carcinog Mutagen, **8**: 377-391.

Evenson DP, Janca FC, & Jost LK (1987) Effects of the fungicide methyl-benzimidazol-2-yl carbamate (MBC) on mouse germ cells as determined by flow cytometry. J Toxicol Environ Health, **20**: 387-399.

Everhart LP (1979) Benlate dust exposure survey. Wilmington, Delaware, E.I. Du Pont de Nemours and Co., Inc. (Unpublished report No. B/TOX 6).

Everhart LP & Holt RF (1982) Potential benlate fungicide exposure during mixer/loader operations, crop harvest and home use. J Agric Food Chem, **30**: 222-227.

Fahrig R & Seiler JP (1979) Dose and effect of methyl 2-benzimidazolyl-carbamate in the "mammalian spot test", an *in vivo* method for the detection of genetic alterations in somatic cells of mice. Chem-Biol Interact, **26**: 115-120.

FAO/WHO (1985a) Benomyl. In: Pesticide residues in food - Evaluations 1983. Rome, Food and Agriculture Organization of the United Nations, pp 7-46 (FAO Plant Production and Protection Paper 61).

FAO/WHO (1985b) Carbendazim. In: Pesticide residues in food - Evaluations 1983. Rome, Food and Agriculture Organization of the United Nations, pp 89-121 (FAO Plant Production and Protection Paper 61).

FAO/WHO (1988a) Benomyl. In: Pesticide residues in food - Evaluations 1988. Part I: Residues. Rome, Food and Agriculture Organization of the United Nations, pp 5-15 (FAO Plant Production and Protection Paper 93/1).

FAO/WHO (1988b) Carbendazim. In: Pesticide residues in food - Evaluations 1988. Part I: Residues. Rome, Food and Agriculture Organization of the United Nations, pp 41-54 (FAO Plant Production and Protection Paper 93/1).

Fielding M, Barcelo D, Helweg A, Galassi S, Torstensson L, van Zoonen P, Wolter R, & Angeletti G (1992) Pesticides in ground and drinking water. Brussels, Commission of the European Communities, Directorate-General for Science, Research and Development, Environment and Waste Recycling, 135 pp (Water Pollution Research Report 27).

Fink R (1975) Eight-day dietary $LC_{50}$ - Mallard ducks. Sterling, Virginia, Truslow Farms, Inc. (Unpublished report No. HLO 108-75, prepared for E.I. Du Pont de Nemours and Co., Inc.).

Fiscor G, Bordas S, & Steward SJ (1978) Mutagenicity testing of benomyl, methyl-2-benzimidazole carbamate, streptozotocin and N-methyl-N'-nitro-N-nitrosoguanine in *Salmonella typhimurium in vitro* and in rodent host-mediated assays. Mutat Res, **51**: 151-164.

Fleeker JR & Lacy HM (1977) Photolysis of methyl 2-benzimidazole-carbamate. J Agric Food Chem, **25**: 51-55.

Ford LS (1981) Primary skin irritation and sensitization on guinea pigs. Newark, Delaware, E.I. Du Pont de Nemours and Co., Inc., Haskell Laboratory (Unpublished report No. HLR 729-81).

Ford LS (1982) Acute skin absorption $LD_{50}$ test on rabbits (carbendazim 75% wettable powder). Newark, Delaware, E.I. Du Pont de Nemours and Co., Inc., Haskell Laboratory (Unpublished report No. HLR 822-81).

Freidman PA & Platzer EG (1978) Interaction of anthelmintic benzimidazoles and benzimidazoles derivatives with bovine brain tubulin. Biochim Biophys Acta, **544**: 605-614.

Galloway SM & Ivett JL (1986) Chemically induced aneuploidy in mammalian cells in culture. Mutat Res, **167**: 89-105.

Gericke D (1977) Test for mutagenicity in bacteria strains in the absence and presence of a liver preparation. Frankfurt, Germany, Hoechst AG, Laboratory for Cancer Research (Report No. A/12202).

Gillet C & Roubaud P (1983) Prehatching survival of carp eggs after treatment during fertilization and early development with the antimitotic fungicide carbendazim. Water Res, **17**: 1343-1348.

Goldenthal EI (1978) Neurotoxicity in hens. Mattawan, Michigan, International Research and Development Corporation (Unpublished report No. HLO 27-79, prepared for E.I. Du Pont de Nemours and Co., Inc.).

Goldman JM, Rehnberg GL, Cooper RL, Gray LE Jr, Hein JF, & McElroy WK (1989) Effects of the benomyl metabolite, carbendazim, on the hypothalamic-pituitary reproductive axis in the male rat. Toxicology, **57**(2): 173-182.

Gooch JJ (1978) Fertility of workers potentially exposed to benomyl. Wilmington, Delaware, E.I. Du Pont de Nemours and Co., Inc. (Unpublished report No. B/TOX 7).

Goodman NC (1974) Intraperitoneal $LD_{50}$ test [in rats using technical carbendazim (less than 98%)]. Newark, Delaware, E.I. Du Pont de Nemours and Co., Inc., Haskell Laboratory (Unpublished report No. HLR 845-74).

Goodman NC & Sherman H (1975) Oral $LD_{50}$ tests (fasted male and female rats). Newark, Delaware, E.I. Du Pont de Nemours and Co., Inc., Haskell Laboratory (Unpublished report No. HLR 847-74).

Grandizio AM & Sarver JW (1987) Acute oral toxicity study with INE-965-261 (Benlate C) in male and female rats. Newark, Delaware, E.I. Du Pont de Nemours and Co., Inc., Haskell Laboratory (Unpublished report No. HLR 358-87).

Gray LE, Ostby J, Sigmon R, Ferrell J, Rehnberg G, Linder R, Cooper R, Goldman J, & Laskey J (1988) The development of a protocol to assess reproductive effects of toxicants in the rat. Reprod Toxicol, **2**: 281-287.

Gray LE, Ostby J, Linder R, Goldman J, Rehnberg G, & Cooper R (1990) Carbendazim-induced alterations of reproductive development and function in the rat and hamster. Fundam Appl Toxicol, **15**: 281-297.

Guengerich FP (1981) Enzyme induction with Du Pont compounds H11,201-02 and H10,962-02. Nashville, Tennessee, Vanderbilt University, School of Medicine (Unpublished report No. HLO-850-81, prepared for E.I. Du Pont de Nemours and Co., Inc.).

Gupta VK & Sharma SD (1989) Degradation of carbendazim in soil by microorganisms. Indian J Agric Sci, **59**: 21-24.

Gustafson DI (1989) Groundwater ubiquity score: A simple method for assessing pesticide leachability. Environ Toxicol Chem, **8**: 339-357.

Hammerschlag RS & Sisler HD (1973) Benomyl and methyl-2-benzimidazole (MBC): biochemical, cytological, and chemical aspects of toxicity to *Ustilage maydis* and *Saccharomyces cerevesiae*. Pestic Biochem Physiol, **3**: 42-54.

Han JC-Y (1983a) Characterization of residues in bean plants following foliar spray applications with methyl 2-$^{14}$C-benzimidazolecarbamate (MBC). Wilmington, Delaware, E.I. Du Pont de Nemours and Co., Inc. (Unpublished report No. MBC/ME-4).

Han JC-Y (1983b) Anaerobic soil metabolism of 2-$^{14}$C-benomyl and methyl 2-$^{14}$C-benzimidazolecarbamate. Wilmington, Delaware, E.I. Du Pont de Nemours and Co., Inc. (Unpublished report No. B/ME-44).

Heinemann JM (1971) Acute static fish (rainbow trout) toxicity study - freshwater (MBC). Vienna, Virginia, Hazelton Laboratories (Unpublished report No. HLO-150-71, prepared for E.I. Du Pont de Nemours and Co., Inc.).

Helweg A (1977) Degradation and adsorption of carbendazim and 2-aminobenzimidazole in soil. Pestic Sci, **8**: 71-78.

Helweg A (1979) Influence of temperature, humidity, and inoculation on the degradation of $^{14}$C-labelled 2-aminobenzimidazole in soil. Water Air Soil Pollut, **12**: 275-281.

Helweg A (1985) Side effects caused by pesticide combinations. In: Jensen V, Kjøller A, & Sørensen LH ed. Proceedings of the FEMS Symposium on Microbial Communities in Soil. Amsterdam, Oxford, New York, Elsevier Science Publishers, pp 385-395.

Hill EF & Camardese MB (1986) Lethal toxicities of environmental contaminants and pesticides to Coturnix. Washington, DC, US Department of the Interior, Fish and Wildlife Service (Fish and Wildlife Technical Report No. 2).

Hinckle L (1981) Oral $LD_{50}$ test in rats - EPA proposed guidelines. Newark, Delaware, E.I. du Pont de Nemours and Co., Inc., Haskell Laboratory (Unpublished report No. HLR 769-81).

Hoechst (1974) Mouse dominant lethal study on MBC. Frankfurt, Germany, Hoechst AG.

Hofer I, Beck T, & Wallnöfer P (1971) [The influence of the fungicide benomyl on soil microflora.] Z Pflanzenkr Pflanzenschutz, **78**: 399-405 (in German).

Holden HE, Crider PA, & Wahrenburg MG (1980) Mitotic arrest by benzimidazole analogs in human lymphocyte cultures. Environ Mutat, **2**: 67-73.

Hughes DL (1984) Residue study of the fungicide MBC in lactating dairy cattle. Madison, Wisconsin, Hazelton Laboratories America, Inc. (Unpublished report No. AMR 429-85, prepared for E.I. Du Pont de Nemours and Co., Inc.).

Hutton DG (1988) Static acute 48-hours $EC_{50}$ of carbamic acid, 1H-benzimidazol-2-yl-, methyl ester to fed *Daphnia magna*. Newark, Delaware, E.I. Du Pont de Nemours and Co., Inc., Haskell Laboratory (Unpublished report No. HLR 638-88).

Hutton DG, Kasprzak DJ, & Priester TM (1984) Laboratory studies of [2-$^{14}$C] carbendazim bioconcentration in bluegill sunfish. Newark, Delaware, E.I. Du Pont de Nemours and Co., Inc., Haskell Laboratory (Unpublished report No. HLR 428-84).

Hutton DG, Lieder PH, & Grapel GJ (1986) Chronic toxicity of carbamic acid, 1H-benzimidazol-2-yl-, methyl ester to *Daphnia magna*. Newark, Delaware, E.I. Du Pont de Nemours and Co., Inc., Haskell Laboratory (Unpublished report No. HLR 241-86).

ILO (1991) Occupational exposure limits for airborne toxic substances, 3rd ed. Geneva, International Labour Office, 455 pp (Occupational Safety and Health Series No. 37).

Ireland CM, Gull K, Gutteridge WE, & Pogson CI (1979) The interaction of benzimidazole carbamates with mammalian microtubule protein. Biochem Pharmacol, **28**: 2680-2682.

Ivett JL (1984) Mutagenicity evaluation of H#15,152 in an *in vitro* sister chromatid exchange assay in Chinese hamster ovary (CHO) cells. Kensington, Maryland, Litton Bionetics, Inc. (Unpublished report No. HLO 254-84, prepared for E.I. Du Pont de Nemours and Co., Inc.).

Janardhan A, Sattur PB, & Sisodia P (1984) Teratology of methyl benzimidazole carbamate in rats and rabbits. Bull Environ Contam Toxicol, **33**(3): 257-263.

Janardhan A, Rao AB, & Sisodia P (1987) Sub-chronic toxicity of methyl benzimidazole carbamate in rats. Bull Environ Contam Toxicol, **38**(5): 890-898.

Jansz GF & Pomerantz DK (1985) The effect of prenatal treatment with busulfan on *in vitro* androgen production by testes from rats of various ages. Can J Physiol Pharmacol, **63**: 1155-1158.

Johnson JD (1988) Determination of the plateau level of bound [phenyl(U)-$^{14}$C]carbendazim residues in goat liver. Columbus, Ohio, Battelle Columbus Division (Unpublished report No. AMR-779-87, prepared for E.I. Du Pont de Nemours and Co., Inc.).

Jotz MM (1980) An evaluation of mutagenic potential of benomyl employing the L5178Y TK+/- mouse lymphoma assay (SRI Project No. LSU 7558). Menlo Park, California, SRI International (Unpublished report prepared for the US Environmental Protection Agency).

Keogh RG & Whitehead PH (1975) Observations on some effects of pasture spraying with benomyl and carbendazim on earthworm activity and litter removal from pasture. NZ J Exp Agric, **3**: 103-104.

Khan S, Khan NN, & Khan FA (1987) The influence of bavistin and calixin on carbon dioxide-evolution and the major nutrient status (nitrogen, phosphorus, potassium) of the soil. Environ Pollut, **47**(2): 115-122.

Kirkland JJ (1973) Method for high-speed liquid chromatographic analysis of benomyl and/or metabolite residue in cow milk, urine, feces and tissues. J Agric Food Chem, **21**: 171-177.

Kirkland JJ, Holt RF, & Pease HL (1973) Determination of benomyl residues in soils and plant tissues by high-speed cation exchange liquid chromatography. J Agric Food Chem, **21**: 368-371.

Koeter HBWM (1975a) Effect of HOE 17411F (=BAS 3460F) on pregnancy of the rat. The Hague, Central Institute of Nutrition and Food Research (TNO) (Unpublished report No. R-4726, prepared for Hoechst AG, Frankfurt and BASF AG, Ludwigshafen).

Koeter HBWM (1975b) Effect of HOE 17411F (=BAS 3460F) on pregnancy of the New Zealand white rabbit. The Hague, Central Institute for Nutrition and Food Research (TNO) (Unpublished report No. R-4881, prepared for Hoechst AG, Frankfurt and BASF AG, Ludwigshafen).

Kramer M & Weigand W (1971) (HOE 17411 O F) Toxicological examination. Frankfurt, Germany, Hoechst AG, Pharmaceuticals Research, Toxicology Section (Unpublished report No. A-00936).

Krechniak J & Klosowska B (1986) The fate of $^{14}$C-carbendazim in rat. Xenobiotica, **16**(9): 809-815.

Lamb MJ & Lilly LJ (1980) An investigation of some genetic toxicological effects of the fungicide benomyl. Toxicology, **17**: 83-95.

Litton (1981) Evaluation of HOE 17411 O F AT204 in the primary rat hepatocyte unscheduled DNA synthesis assay (LBI Project No. 21001). Kensington, Maryland, Litton Bionetics, Inc. (Unpublished report prepared for Hoechst AG, Frankfurt).

Lofs-Holmin A (1981) Influence in field experiments of benomyl and carbendazim on earthworms (*Lumbricidae*) in relation to soil texture. Swed J Agric Res, **11**: 141-147.

Lofs-Holmin A (1982) Influence of routine pesticide spraying on earthworms (*Lumbricidea*) in field experiments with winter wheat. Swed J Agric Res, **12**: 121-124.

Marsh BH & Arthur MF (1989) Aerobic metabolism of [phenyl(U)-$^{14}$C]benomyl in keyport silt loam. Columbus, Ohio, Battelle Memorial Institute (Unpublished report No. AMR 1112-88, prepared for E.I. Du Pont de Nemours and Co., Inc.).

Martin DA, Henry JE, & Brock WJ (1987) Closed-patch repeated insult dermal sensitization study (Buehler Method) with Benlate C fungicide in guinea-pigs. Newark, Delaware, E.I. Du Pont de Nemours and Co., Inc., Haskell Laboratory (Unpublished report No. HLR 510-87).

Marvin Ch, Birndle ID, Hall CD, & Chiba M (1991) Rapid on-line precolumn high performance liquid chromatographic method for the determination of benomyl, carbendazim and aldicarb species in drinking water. J Chromatogr, **555**: 147-154.

Mayer FL & Ellersieck MR (1986) Manual of acute toxicity: Interpretation and data base for 410 chemicals and 66 species of freshwater animals. Washington, DC, US Department of the Interior, Fish and Wildlife Service, pp 45-46 (Resource Publication No. 160).

Mazur AR & Hughes TD (1975) Nitrogen transformations in soil as affected by the fungicides benomyl, dyrene and maneb. Agron J, **67**: 755-758.

Meade AB (1984) Acute contact $LD_{50}$ toxicity study in honey bees (*Apis mellifera* L.) with INE965-212 (MBC). Wilmington, Delaware, E.I. Du Pont de Nemours and Co., Inc. (Unpublished report No. ABM-84-5).

Mohr U (1977) Review of liver sections from mice and rats fed with carbendazim. Hannover, Germany, Medical School, Department of Experimental Pathology (Unpublished report No. MBC/TOX 6, prepared for Hoechst AG, Frankfurt and BASF AG, Ludwigshafen).

Monson KD (1985) Metabolism of [2-$^{14}$C]-carbendazim in the lactating dairy cow. Wilmington, Delaware, E.I. Du Pont de Nemours and Co., Inc. (Unpublished report No. AMR 248-84).

Monson KD (1986) Metabolism of [2-$^{14}$C]-carbendazim in laying hens. Wilmington, Delaware, E.I. Du Pont de Nemours and Co., Inc. (Unpublished report No. AMR 264-84).

Monson KD (1990) Metabolism of [phenyl(U)-$^{14}$C]carbendazim in rats. Wilmington, Delaware, E.I. Du Pont de Nemours and Co., Inc. (Unpublished report No. AMR-1141-88).

Monson KD (1991) Release and characterization of bound benomyl and carbendazim metabolites in animal tissues via Raney nickel desulfurization and acid dehydration. J Agric Food Chem, **39**: 1808-1811.

Nakai M, Hess RA, Moore BJ, Guttroff RF, Strader LF, & Linder RE (1992) Acute and long-term effects of a single dose of the fungicide carbendazim (methyl 2-benzimidazole carbamate) on the male reproductive system in the rat. J Androl, **13**: 507-518.

Nash SD & Ferenz R (1982) Inhalation median lethal concentration ($LC_{50}$ in rats -EPA protocol (carbendazim 75% wettable powder). Newark, Delaware, E.I. Du Pont de Nemours and Co., Inc., Haskell Laboratory (Unpublished report No. HLR 365-82).

Newsome WH & Collins PG (1987) Enzyme-linked immunosorbent assay of benomyl and thiabendazole in some foods. J Assoc Off Anal Chem, **70**: 1025-1027.

Newsome WH & Shields JB (1981) A radioimmunoassay for benomyl and methyl 2-benzimidazolecarbamate on food. J Agric Food Chem, **29**: 220-222.

Nishiuchi Y & Yoshida K (1974) Toxicity of new agricultural chemicals to tadpoles. Bull Agric Chem Insp Stn, **14**: 66-68.

Osgood C, Zimmering S, & Mason JM (1991) Aneuploidy in Drosophila. II. Further validation of the FIX and ZESTE genetic test systems employing female *Drosophila melanogaster*. Mutat Res, **259**: 147-163.

Palawski DU & Knowles CO (1986) Toxicological studies of benomyl and carbendazim in rainbow trout, channel catfish and bluegills. Environ Toxicol Chem, **5**: 1039-1046.

Pandita TK (1988) Assessment of the mutagenic potential of a fungicide Bavistin using multiple assays. Mutat Res, **204**: 627-643.

Parsons DW & Witt JM (1988) Pesticides in groundwater in the United States of America: A report of a 1988 survey of State lead agencies. Corvallis, Oregon, Oregon State University Extension Service.

Peeples JL (1974) Microbial activity in benomyl-treated soil. Phytopathology, **64**: 857-860.

Perreault SD, Jeffay S, Poss P, & Laskey JW (1992) Use of the fungicide carbendazim as a model compound to determine the impact of acute chemical exposure during oocyte maturation and fertilization on pregnancy outcome in the hamster. Toxicol Appl Pharmacol, **114**: 225-231.

Priester TM (1984) Hydrolysis of carbendazim [2-$^{14}$C]. Newark, Delaware, E.I. Du Pont de Nemours and Co., Inc., Haskell Laboratory (Unpublished report No. AMR 265-84).

Purser D (1987) Carbendazim: behaviour in water. Harrogate, North Yorkshire, United Kingdom, Hazelton Laboratories (Unpublished report No. 5220-269/12, prepared for E.I. Du Pont de Nemours and Co., Inc.).

Ramakrishna C, Gowda TKS, & Sethunathan N (1979) Effect of benomyl and its hydrolysis products, MBC and AB on nitrification in flooded soil. Bull Environ Contam Toxicol, **21**: 328-333.

Rashid MA & Mumma RO (1986) Screening pesticides for their availability to damage bacterial DNA. J Environ Sci Health, **B21**: 319-334.

Raw F (1962) Studies of earthworm populations in orchards. Ann Appl Biol, **50**: 389-404.

Rehnberg GL, Cooper RL, Goldman JM, Gray LE, Hein JF, & McElroy WK (1989) Serum and testicular testosterone and androgen binding protein profiles following subchronic treatment with carbendazim. Toxicol Appl Pharmacol, **101**: 55-61.

Reuzel PGJ, Hendriksen CFM, & Til HP (1976) Long-term (two-year) toxicity study with carbendazim in beagle dogs. The Hague, Central Institute for Nutrition and Food Research (TNO) (Unpublished report prepared for BASF AG, Ludwigshafen and Hoechst AG, Frankfurt).

Rhodes RC (1987) Greenhouse crop-rotation study with [2-$^{14}$C]carbendazim. Wilmington, Delaware, E.I. Du Pont de Nemours and Co., Inc. (Unpublished report No. AMR-495-86).

Rhodes RC & Long JD (1983) Run-off and leaching studies with methyl 2-$^{14}$C-benzimidazolecarbamate on soil. Wilmington, Delaware, E.I. Du Pont de Nemours and Co., Inc. (Unpublished report No. MBC/ME-9).

Rhodes RC, Pease HL, & Holt RF (1983) Greenhouse studies on crop uptake of MBC and 2-AB from soil. Wilmington, Delaware, E.I. Du Pont de Nemours and Co., Inc. (Unpublished Report No. MBC/ME-5).

Roberts BL & Dorough HW (1984) Relative toxicities on chemicals to the earthworm *Eisenia foetida*. Environ Toxicol Chem, **3**: 67-78.

Russel LD, Ettlin RA, Sinha Hikim AP, & Clegg ER (1990) Histological and histopathological evaluation of the testis. Clearwater, Florida, Cache River Press.

Russell JF (1977) Mutagenicity evaluation of 2-benzimidazolecarbamic acid, 5-hydroxy-, methyl in *Salmonella typhimurium*. Newark, Delaware, E.I. Du Pont de Nemours and Co., Inc., Haskell Laboratory (Unpublished report).

Russell JF (1983) Mutagenicity evaluation in *Salmonella typhimurium*. Newark, Delaware, E.I. Du Pont de Nemours and Co., Inc., Haskell Laboratory (Unpublished report No. HLR 179-83).

Sarver JW (1975) Acute inhalation toxicity - one hour head only (carbendazim). Newark, Delaware, E.I. Du Pont de Nemours and Co., Inc., Haskell Laboratory (Unpublished report No. HLR 58-75).

Scholz J & Weigand W (1972) Carbendazim (HOE 17411 O F, batch 496/I). Toxicological examination. Frankfurt, Germany, Hoechst AG, Pharmaceuticals Research, Toxicology Section (Unpublished report No. A-00935).

Seiler JP (1976) The mutagenicity of benzimidazole and benzimidazole derivatives. VI. Cytogenetic effects of benzimidazole derivatives in the bone marrow of the mouse and the Chinese hamster. Mutat Res, **40**: 339-348.

Seiler JP (1977) Apparent and real thresholds: A study on two mutagens. In: Scott D, Bridges BA, & Sobels FH ed. Progress in genetic toxicology. Amsterdam, Elsevier/North-Holland Biomedical Press, pp 233-238.

Sheir-Neiss F, Nardi RV, Gealt A, & Morris NR (1976) Tubulin-like protein from *Aspergillus nidulans*. Biochem Biophys Res Commun, **69**: 285-290.

Sherman H (1965) Acute oral test. Newark, Delaware, E.I. Du Pont de Nemours and Co., Inc., Haskell Laboratory (Unpublished report No. HLR 125-65).

Sherman H (1968) Ninety-day feeding study in rats using a wettable powder formulation (70% MBC). Newark, Delaware, E.I. Du Pont de Nemours and Co., Inc., Haskell Laboratory (Unpublished report No. HLR 95-68).

Sherman H (1970) Three-month feeding study in dogs using a wettable powder formulation (50% MBC). Newark, Delaware, E.I. Du Pont de Nemours and Co., Inc., Haskell Laboratory (Unpublished report No. HLR 283-70).

Sherman H (1972) Long-term feeding studies in rats and dogs with 2-benzimadazole-carbamic acid, methyl ester (INE-965) (50% and 70% MBC wettable powder formulations). Parts I and II. Newark, Delaware, E.I. Du Pont de Nemours and Co., Inc., Haskell Laboratory (Unpublished report No. HLR 195-72).

Sherman H & Krauss WC (1966) Acute oral test (carbendazim). Newark, Delaware, E.I. Du Pont de Nemours and Co., Inc., Haskell Laboratory (Unpublished report No. HLR 99-66).

Sheu CW, Lee JK, Arras CA, Jones RL, & Lavappa KS (1990) The feasibility of using Chinese hamster as an animal model for aneuploidy. Environ Mol Mutagen, **16**: 320-323.

Shirasu Y, Moriya M, & Kato K (1977) Mutagenicity testing on fungicide 1991 in microbial systems. Tokyo, Institute of Environmental Toxicology, Kodaira Laboratories (Unpublished report prepared for E.I. Du Pont de Nemours and Co., Inc.).

Shukla Y, Antony M, & Mehrotra NK (1989) Studies on g-glutamyl transpeptidase in rodents exposed to benomyl. Bull Environ Contam Toxicol, **42**: 301-306.

Siebert D, Zimmermann FK, & Lemperle E (1970) Genetic effects of fungicides. Mutat Res, **10**: 533-543.

Speakman JB & Nirenberg HI (1981) Mutagenicity of methyl benzimidazole-2-yl carbamate (MBC) towards *Aspergillus nidulans* (Eidam) Winter and *Cladosporium cucumerinum* Ellis and Arth. Mutat Res, **88**: 45-51.

Stadler JC (1986) One-year feeding study in dogs with carbendazim. Newark, Delaware, E.I. Du Pont de Nemours and Co., Inc., Haskell Laboratory (Unpublished report No. HLR 291-86).

Staub T & Sozzi D (1984) Fungicide resistance: A continuing challenge. Plant Dis, **68**: 1026-1031.

Stringer A & Lyons C (1974) The effect of benomyl and thiophanate-methyl on earthworm populations in apple orchards. Pestic Sci, **5**: 189-196.

Stringer A & Wright MA (1973) The effect of benomyl and some related compounds on *Lumbricus terrestris* and other earthworms. Pestic Sci, **4**: 165-170.

Styles JA & Garner R (1974) Benzimidazolecarbamate methyl ester - evaluation of its effects *in vivo* and *in vitro*. Mutat Res, **26**: 177-187.

Til HP, van den Muelen HC, Feron VJ, Seinen W, & de Groot AP (1972) Sub-chronic (90-day) toxicity study with W17411 in beagle dogs. The Hague, Central Institute for Nutrition and Food Research (TNO) (Unpublished report No. R-3920, prepared for Hoechst AG, Frankfurt).

Til HP, Koellen C, & van der Heijden CA (1976a) Combined chronic toxicity and carcinogenicity study with carbendazim in rats. The Hague, Central Institute for Nutrition and Food Research (TNO) (Unpublished report prepared for BASF AG, Ludwigshafen and Hoechst AG, Frankfurt).

Til HP, Koeter HBWM, & van der Heijden CA (1976b) Multigeneration study with carbendazim in rats. The Hague, Central Institute for Nutrition and Food Research (TNO) (Unpublished report No. R-5024, prepared for Hoechst AG, Frankfurt).

Til HP, Beems RB, & de Groot AP (1981) Determination of the acute oral toxicity of carbendazim in mice. The Hague, Central Institute for Nutrition and Food Research (TNO) (Unpublished report No. A-21604, prepared for BASF AG, Ludwigshafen).

Tong C (198la) Hepatocyte primary culture/DNA repair assay on compound 11, 201-01 (MBC) using mouse hepatocytes in culture. Valhalla, New York, Naylor Dana Institute (Unpublished report No. HLO 743-81, prepared for E.I. Du Pont de Nemours and Co., Inc.).

Tong C (198lb) Hepatocyte primary culture/DNA repair assay on compound 11,201-01 (MBC) using rat hepatocytes in culture. Valhalla, New York, Naylor Dana Institute (Unpublished report No. HLO 744-81, prepared for E.I. Du Pont de Nemours and Co., Inc.).

Torstensson L & Wessen B (1984) Interactions between the fungicide benomyl and soil microorganisms. Soil Biol Biochem, **16**: 445-452.

Van Faassen HG (1974) Effect of the fungicide benomyl on some metabolic processes and on numbers of bacteria and actinomycetes in the soil. Soil Biol Biochem, **6**: 131-133.

Van Gestel CAM (1992) Validation of earthworm toxicity tests by comparison with field studies: A review of benomyl, carbendazim, carbofuran, and carbaryl. Ecotoxicol Environ Saf, **23**: 221-236.

Van Gestel CAM, Dirven-van Breeman EM, Baerselman R, Emans HJB, Janssen JAM, Postuma R, & van Vliet PJM (1992) Comparison of sublethal and lethal criteria for nine different chemicals in standardized toxicity tests using the earthworm *Eisenia andrei*. Ecotoxicol Environ Saf, **23**: 206-220.

Vick DA & Brock WJ (1987a) Primary dermal irritation study with Benlate C fungicide in rabbits. Newark, Delaware, E.I. Du Pont de Nemours and Co., Inc., Haskell Laboratory (Unpublished report No. HLR 299-87).

Vick DA & Brock WJ (1987b) Acute dermal toxicity study of Benlate C fungicide in rabbits. Newark, Delaware, E.I. Du Pont de Nemours and Co., Inc., Haskell Laboratory (Unpublished report No. HLR 303-87).

Vick DA & Valentine R (1987) Primary eye irritation study with Benlate C fungicide in rabbits. Newark, Delaware, E.I. Du Pont de Nemours and Co., Inc., Haskell Laboratory (Unpublished report No. HLR 287-87).

Vonk JW, Adema OMM, & Barug D (1986) Comparison of the effects of several chemicals on microorganisms, higher plants and earthworms. In: Assink JW & van den Brink WG ed. Contaminated soil. Dordrecht, Boston, Lancaster, Martinus Nijhoff Publishers, p 191.

Wainwright M & Pugh GJF (1974) The effect of fungicides on certain chemical and microbial properties of soils. Soil Biol Biochem, **6**: 263-267.

Wallin M, Friden B, & Billger M (1989) Studies of the interaction of chemicals with microtubule assembly *in vitro* can be used as an assay for detection of cytotoxic chemicals and possible inducers of aneuploidy. Mutat Res, **201**: 303-311.

Waterer JC (1980) Chinese hamster ovary cell assay for mutagenicity. Newark, Delaware, E.I. Du Pont de Nemours and Co., Inc., Haskell Laboratory (Unpublished report No. HLR 660-88).

Weeks RE & Hedrick HG (1975) Influence of a systemic fungicide on oxygen uptake by soil microorganisms. Soil Sci, **119**: 280-284.

Wetzel JW & Hutton DG (1984) 96-Hour $LC_{50}$ to bluegill sunfish. Newark, Delaware, E.I. Du Pont de Nemours and Co., Inc., Haskell Laboratory (Unpublished report No. HLR 401-84).

Whittaker SG, Moser SF, Maloney DH, Piegorsch WW, Resnick MA, & Fogel S (1990) The detection of mitotic and meiotic chromosome gain in the yeast *Saccharomyces cerevisiae*: Effects of methyl benzimidazol-2-yl carbamate, methyl methanesulfonate, ethyl methanesulfonate, dimethyl sulfoxide, propionitrile and cyclophosphamide monohydrate. Mutat Res, **242**: 231-258.

WHO (1993) Environmental Health Criteria 148: Benomyl. Geneva, World Health Organization.

Wood CK (1982) Long-term feeding study with 2-benzimidazole-carbamate, methyl ester (< 99% MBC, INE-965) in mice. Parts I and II. Newark, Delaware, E.I. Du Pont de Nemours and Co., Inc., Haskell Laboratory (Unpublished report No. HLR 70-82).

Yarden O, Aharonson N, & Katan J (1987) Accelerated microbial degradation of methyl benzimidizol-2-ylcarbamate in soil and its control. Soil Biol Biochem, **19**(6): 735-739.

# RESUME ET CONCLUSIONS

## 1. Résumé

### 1.1 Identité, propriétés physiques et chimiques et méthodes d'analyse

Le carbendazime, un solide cristallin blanc, est un fongicide endothérapique qui appartient à la famille du benzimidazole. Son point de fusion est d'environ 250 °C et sa tension de vapeur est $< 1 \times 10^{-7}$ Pa ($< 1 \times 10^{-9}$ mbar) à 20 °C. Le carbendazime est pratiquement insoluble dans l'eau, sa solubilité n'étant que de 8 mg/litre à pH 7 et à 20 °C. Il est stable dans les conditions normales de stockage.

L'analyse des résidus de même que celle des prélèvements effectués dans l'environnement comportent une extraction au moyen d'un solvant organique et une purification de l'extrait par partage liquide-liquide. Le dosage de ces résidus peut s'effectuer par chromatographie en phase liquide à haute performance ou par titrage immunologique.

### 1.2 Sources d'exposition humaine et environnementale

Le carbendazime est, parmi les fongicides de la famille du benzimidazole, celui qui est le plus largement utilisé. Il est présenté sous forme de dispersion ou de suspension aqueuse, de granulés fluants dispersables dans l'eau et de poudre mouillable.

### 1.3 Transport, distribution et transformation dans l'environnement

Le carbendazime est d'ailleurs le produit de transformation dans l'environnement du bénomyl, un autre fongicide benzimidazolique; la réaction est rapide avec une demi-vie respective de 2 et 19 heures dans l'eau et le sol. On peut donc utiliser les résultats des études sur le bénomyl ou sur le carbendazime pour l'évaluation des effets sur l'environnement.

Dans l'environnement, le carbendazime se décompose avec une demi-vie de 6 à 12 mois sur le sol nu, de 3 à 6 mois sur le gazon et de 2 à 25 mois dans l'eau en aérobiose et en anaérobiose, respectivement. Le carbendazime est principalement décomposé par les microorganismes. Le 2-aminobenzimidazole (2-AB) en est l'un des principaux produits de dégradation et il est à son tour décomposé par les microorganismes. Lors de la décomposition du bénomyl marqué au $^{14}C$ sur le noyau phényle, on a constaté que 9% seulement du carbone-14 était éliminé sous forme de $CO_2$ en une année d'incubation. Le carbone-14 restant était principalement récupéré sous forme de carbendazime et de résidus liés. L'étude de la destinée d'un éventuel produit de dégradation (1,2-diamino-benzène) pourrait peut-être permettre de mieux définir la voie de dégradation des fongicides benzimidazoliques dans l'environnement.

Des études effectuées sur le terrain ou sur colonne ont montré que le carbendazime restait dans les couches superficielles du sol. On n'a pas mesuré l'adsorption du carbendazime dans le sol, mais on pense qu'elle doit être aussi forte que dans le cas du bénomyl, avec des valeurs de $K_{oc}$ allant de 1000 à 3600. Les valeurs de log $K_{ow}$ sont respectivement de 1,36 et de 1,49 pour le bénomyl et le carbendazime.

Un modèle de criblage basé sur les données d'adsorption et de persistance n'a pas révélé de risque de lessivage. Cette observation est corroborée par des analyses d'eau de pluie effectuées aux Etats-Unis, analyses qui n'ont pas permis de déceler ce composé dans l'un quelconque des 212 puits étudiés (la limite de détection n'a pas été précisée). On estime que le bénomyl et le carbendazime entraînés par ruissellement correspondent uniquement à la fraction adsorbée aux particules de sol; d'ailleurs ces composés sont sans doute fortement adsorbés aux sédiments présents dans l'environnement aquatique.

Le carbendazime est hydrolysé en 2-AB. Ce produit en constitue également le principal métabolite dans le sol et les végétaux.

Chez l'animal, le carbendazime est métabolisé en (5-hydroxy-1H-benzimidazole-2-yl)-carbamate (5-HBC) et autres métabolites polaires, qui sont rapidement excrétés. On n'a pas observé d'accumulation de carbendazime dans aucun système biologique.

### 1.4 Concentrations dans l'environnement et exposition humaine

Il ne semble pas qu'il existe de données résultant d'une surveillance du carbendazime dans l'environnement. Toutefois on peut récapituler comme suit les données d'études portant sur la destinée écologique de ce produit.

Comme le bénomyl et le carbendazime restent stable pendant des semaines sur les végétaux, ils peuvent être ingérés par des organismes qui se nourrissent de feuilles mortes. Des résidus de carbendazime peuvent subsister jusqu'à 3 ans dans le sol et les sédiments. Toutefois la forte adsorption du carbendazime aux particules de sol et de sédiments réduit l'exposition des organismes terrestres et aquatiques.

Ce sont les résidus de bénomyl et de carbendazime présents sur les cultures vivrières qui constituent la principale source d'exposition de la population humaine dans son ensemble. L'analyse de l'exposition par voie alimentaire qui a été effectuée aux Etats-Unis (bénomyl plus carbendazime) et aux Pays-Bas (carbendazime seul) a montré que la quantité moyenne ingérée était vraisemblablement de l'ordre d'une dixième de la dose journalière acceptable (DJA) qui est, pour le bénomyl, de 0.02 mg/kg de poids corporel et pour le carbendazime, de 0,01 mg/kg de poids corporel.

L'exposition professionnelle au cours de la production est inférieure à la valeur-seuil établie pour le bénomyl. Les ouvriers agricoles qui préparent les mélanges, effectuent le remplissage ou retournent dans les champs traités par du bénomyl ou du carbendazime, courent un risque d'exposition cutanée correspondant à quelques milligrammes de bénomyl par heure. Le port de dispositifs de protection permettrait de réduire encore cette exposition. En outre, étant donné que l'absorption percutanée est vraisemblablement faible, il est très peu probable que le carbendazime puisse avoir des effets toxiques généraux sur les populations humaines en étant absorbé par cette voie.

### 1.5 Cinétique et métabolisme

Le carbendazime est bien absorbé (à hauteur de 80 à 85%) après ingestion mais il l'est beaucoup moins après exposition par voie cutanée. Une fois absorbé, le carbendazime donne naissance dans l'organisme à de nombreux métabolites. Les principaux d'entre eux sont le 5-HBC et les 5,6-HOBC-N-oxydes. Le 5,6-DHBC-S et le 5,6-DHBC-G constituent des métabolites mineurs.

D'après la distribution tissulaire du carbendazime, il n'y a pas de bioconcentration. Chez le rat, la concentration la plus élevée après administration par voie orale (< 1% de la dose), a été constatée dans le foie. Le produit se retrouvait sous forme de carbendazime dans les mitochondries, de 5-HBC dans le cytosol et de 2-AB dans les microsomes. On a également retrouvé le carbendazime et ses métabolites dans les reins de poulets et de vaches après exposition, mais il ne se trouvait pas dans les autres tissus en quantités appréciables. Après administration de carbendazime à des vaches laitières, on a retrouvé de petites quantités de 5-HBC et de 4-HBC dans le lait.

Soixante-douze heures après avoir été administré par voie orale à des rats, le carbendazime était excrété dans leurs urines.

Chez les rats et les souris, de fortes doses de carbendazime administrées, soit mêlées à la nourriture, soit par gavage, ont eu un effet sur certaines enzymes microsomiques du foie. Ainsi il y a eu induction de la styrène-7,8-hydrolase et de l'époxyde-hydrolase mais réduction de l'activité de la 7-hydroxycoumarine-O-déséthylase. On a également constaté une induction de l'activité de la glutation-S-transférase du cytosol.

## 1.6 Effets sur les mammifères de laboratoire et sur les systèmes d'épreuve in vitro

### 1.6.1 *Exposition unique*

Le carbendazime présente une faible toxicité aiguë. Les valeurs de la $DL_{50}$ vont de > 2000 à 15 000 mg/kg chez toutes sortes d'animaux d'expérience exposés par diverses voies. Toutefois on n'a pas noté, après exposition unique, d'effets nocifs sensibles sur la reproduction (voir Section 1.6.5).

### 1.6.2 *Exposition de brève durée*

Administré en mélange à la nourriture pendant des périodes allant jusqu'à 90 jours, le carbendazime a entraîné une légère modification du poids du foie chez des rattes qui en avaient reçu une dose quotidienne de 360 mg/kg de poids corporel. Une étude de 90 jours au cours de laquelle du carbendazime a été administré par gavage à des rats, a permis de fixer à 16 mg/kg/jour la dose sans effets observables, basée sur l'hépatotoxicité. Les études d'alimentation de courte durée effectuées sur des chiens se sont révélées insuffisantes pour l'établissement d'une dose sans effets observables. Une étude de 10 jours, au cours de laquelle de lapins ont été exposés au carbendazime par voir cutanée n'a pas permis de mettre en évidence une toxicité générale à la seule dose étudiée (200 mg/kg).

### 1.6.3 Irritation et sensibilisation au niveau de la peau et des yeux

L'application du produit sur l'épiderme de lapins ou de cobayes n'a produit aucune irritation ni sensibilisation de la peau. Chez le lapin, l'instillation oculaire n'a produit qu'une irritation légère à modérée de la conjonctive.

### 1.6.4 Exposition de longue durée

A l'issue d'une étude d'alimentation où des rats mâles et femelles avaient reçu 2500 mg de carbendazime/kg de nourriture, on a constaté une réduction du nombre des érythrocytes ainsi que du taux d'hémoglobine et de l'hématocrite. Aucun effet toxique sur le foie n'a été constaté. Parmi les rats mâles qui avaient reçu du carbendazime à raison de 2500 mg ou davantage/kg de nourriture, on notait une augmentation peu importante du nombre de cas d'atrophie testiculaire diffuse et de prostatite. Chez le rat, la dose sans effets observables est de 500 mg/kg de nourriture. Des chiens qui avaient reçu pendant une année ou davantage une nourriture contenant 500 mg de carbendazime/kg, ont présenté une élévation du taux de cholestérol sérique et de l'activité de la phosphatase alcaline accompagnée d'autres indices d'une hépatotoxicité. Chez le chien, la dose sans effets observables a été fixée à 300 mg/kg de nourriture.

Chez des souris mâles et femelles qui avaient reçu une nourriture contenant 5000 mg de carbendazime/kg de nourriture on a observé une augmentation du poids absolu du foie. Chez des souris mâles ayant reçu 1500 mg de carbendazime/kg de nourriture on a également observé une importante hypertrophie centrilobulaire avec nécrose et hypertrophie générale du foie.

### 1.6.5 Reproduction, embryotoxicité et tératogénicité

Lors d'une étude de reproduction portant sur trois générations, on a administré à des rats du carbendazime à des doses allant jusqu'à 500 mg/kg de nourriture inclusivement; aucun effet nocif n'a été constaté sur la reproduction de ces animaux. En revanche, après administration du même produit par gavage pendant 85 jour à raison de 200 mg/kg/jour, on constatait une réduction de la fertilité des mâles. A la dose de 50 mg/kg de poids corporel, la même étude a révélé une réduction sensible du nombre de spermatozoïdes épididymaires.

Après administration par voie orale d'une dose unique de carbendazime et examen histologique, on a constaté que dès les deux premiers jours, il y avait une forte perturbation de la spermatogénèse avec occlusion des canaux efférents et augmentation du poids des testicules à la dose de 100 mg/kg de poids corporel. Aucun effet n'a été observé au cours de la même étude à la dose de 50 mg/kg. Ces effets ont persisté jusqu'au 70ème jour chez les rats ayant reçu 400 mg/kg.

Administré à des rats en doses quotidiennes supérieures à 10 mg/kg du 7ème au 16ème jour de la gestation, le carbendazime a provoqué une augmentation du nombre de malformations et d'anomalies chez le rat. On constatait également une légère diminution du taux de nidation chez des lapines qui en avaient reçu respectivement 20 ou 125 mg/kg en doses quotidiennes du 7ème au 19ème jour de la gestation ainsi qu'un accroissement de la fréquence des résorptions à la dose quotidienne de 125 mg/kg. Le composé s'est révélé toxique pour la mère, chez la ratte, à la dose quotidienne de 20 mg/kg et chez la lapine à la dose quotidienne de 125 mg/kg.

Outre que le taux de gravidité était en diminution et que la fréquence des résorptions précoces était en augmentation chez le rat, il y avait une réduction sensible du poids des foetus aux doses quotidiennes respectives de 20 et 90 mg/kg, et un accroissement également notable des malformations à la dose quotidienne de 90 mg/kg. Il s'agissait essentiellement d'hydrocéphalie, de microphthalmie, d'anophthalmie, de malformations des omoplates et de la partie axiale du squelette (fusions vertébrales, costales et sternébrales, exencéphalie, hémivertèbres et hyperplasie costale). Toutefois on n'a pas constaté de malformations importantes chez le lapin.

### 1.6.6 *Mutagénicité et autres points d'aboutissement des effets toxiques*

Les épreuves effectuées *in vitro* et *in vivo* sur des systèmes mammaliens et non-mammaliens ainsi que sur des cellules somatiques ou germinales montrent que le carbendazime n'interagit pas avec l'ADN, qu'il ne provoque pas de mutations ponctuelles et ne cause pas de mutation des cellules germinales.

Toutefois le carbendazime provoque des aberrations dans le nombre des chromosomes (aneuploïdie et/ou polyloïdie) dans les systèmes d'épreuve (tant *in vitro* qu'*in vivo*).

### 1.6.7 Cancérogénicité

L'administration de bénomyl et de carbendazime mêlés à la nourriture a provoqué chez des souris CD-1 et Swiss axéniques une augmentation dans l'incidence des tumeurs hépatocellulaires.

Une étude de cancérogénicité a été effectuée avec le carbendazime sur des souris CD-1; elle a révélé une augmentation statistiquement significative et liée à la dose dans l'incidence des néoplasmes hépatocellulaires chez les femelles. Il y avait également une augmentation statistiquement significative à la dose moyenne (1500 mg/kg) de ces anomalies chez les mâles, augmentation qui n'a pas été constatée aux doses élevées en raison du taux élevé de mortalité. Une autre étude de cancérogénicité portant sur le carbendazime a été effectuée chez une souche génétiquement apparentée de souris Swiss axéniques et exogames à des doses de 0, 150, 300 et 1000 mg/kg (la dernière dose étant portée 5000 mg/kg au cours de l'étude); elle a révélé un accroissement dans l'incidence de l'ensemble de adénomes et carcinomes hépatocellulaires. Une troisième étude, effectuée cette fois sur des souris NMRKf à des doses respectives de 0, 50, 150, 300 et 1000 mg/kg de nourriture (la dernière dose étant également portée à 5000 mg/kg au cours de l'étude) n'a cette fois pas fait ressortir d'effets cancérogènes. Le bénomyl ou le carbendazime ont provoqué indifféremment des tumeurs hépatiques chez deux souches de souris (CD-1 et axéniques), souches qui présentent toutes deux un taux élevé de tumeurs hépatiques spontanées. En revanche, le carbendazime n'est pas cancérogène chez les souris NMRKf dont le taux de tumeurs spontanées du foie est faible.

Les études de cancérogénicité portant sur le bénomyl et le carbendazime ont donné des résultats négatifs chez le rat.

### 1.6.8 Mécanisme de la toxicité - mode d'action

On pense que les effets biologiques du bénomyl et du carbendazime résultent de leur interaction avec les microtubules cellulaires. Ces structures interviennent dans des fonctions aussi importantes que la division cellulaire, qui est inhibée par ces deux substances. La toxicité du bénomyl et du carbendazime pour les mammifères est donc liée à une perturbation des fonctions du système microtubulaire.

Comme les autres dérivés du benzimidazole, le bénomyl et le carbendazime sont plus ou moins toxiques selon les espèces. Cette sélectivité toxicologique s'explique au moins en partie par le fait que les deux substances ne se lient pas de la même manière aux tubulines des espèces visées et des espèces non-visées.

### 1.7 Effets sur l'homme

Aucun effet nocif pour la santé humaine n'a été signalé.

### 1.8 Effets sur les autres êtres vivants, en laboratoire et dans leur milieu naturel

Le carbendazime n'a guère d'effet sur l'activité microbienne du sol aux doses d'emploi recommandées. On a cependant signalé l'existence d'effets nocifs vis-à-vis de certains groupes de champignons.

On a calculé que la $CE_{50}$ à 72 heures, fondée sur la croissance totale, pour les algues bleu-vert du genre *Selenastrum capricornutum*, était égale à 1,3 mg/litre; la concentration sans effets observables était de 0,5 mg/litre. La toxicité du carbendazime pour les invertébrés aquatiques et les poissons varie largement, les valeurs de la $CL_{50}$ à 96 heures allant de 0,007 mg/litre pour des poissons chats du genre *Ictalurus*, à 5,5 mg/litre pour *Lepomis machrochirus*. Une étude de 21 jours sur la daphnie *Daphnia magna*, a révélé que, à la dose de 0,025 mg/litre, le déclenchement de la reproduction était sensiblement retardé; la concentration sans effets observables a été fixée à 0,013 mg/litre dans ce cas.

Le carbendazime se montre toxique pour les lombrics dans des expériences de laboratoire reproduisant les conditions réelles d'exposition qui résultent d'une utilisation dans les conditions recommandées sur le terrain. Il est "relativement non toxique" pour les abeilles et peu toxique pour les oiseaux.

## 2. Conclusions

Le bénomyl, un composé voisin du carbendazime, provoque une sensibilisation cutanée chez l'homme. Ce composé et le carbendazime lui-même ne présentent guère de risques d'intoxication aiguë pour l'homme. Etant donné les conditions actuelles d'exposition et le faible taux d'absorption percutanée de ces deux composés, il est improbable qu'ils provoquent des effets toxiques généralisés dans la population ou chez les personnes exposées pour des raisons professionnelles. Ces conclusions résultent des données relatives à l'animal et dans une moindre mesure des données relatives à l'homme; elles reposent sur la connaissance du mode d'action du carbendazime et du bénomyl, tant chez les espèces visées que chez les autres.

Grâce à une meilleure connaissance du mécanisme de la toxicité du bénomyl et du carbendazime chez les mammifères, on pourra peut-être mieux déterminer quelles sont les doses sans effets observables. Des études portant sur la liaison de ces composés aux tubulines des cellules cibles (tissus testiculaires et embryonnaires) faciliteront sans doute les comparaisons interspécifiques.

Le carbendazime est fortement adsorbé aux matières organiques du sol et il y persiste pendant des périodes allant jusqu'à trois ans. Il persiste également sur le feuillage et se retrouve par conséquent dans les feuilles mortes. On a montré que les lombrics pouvaient souffrir (dans leur effectif comme dans leur reproduction) de l'action de ces composés aux doses d'emploi recommandées. On ne possède aucune données sur les autres arthropodes qui vivent dans le sol ou sur les débris organiques et qui pourraient être exposés de la même manière.

Il est improbable que la forte toxicité que, selon les études de la laboratoire, le carbendazime présente pour les organismes aquatiques, s'observe également dans le milieu naturel, du fait de la faible biodisponibilité des résidus de ce composé liés aux sédiments. Toutefois on ne possède aucune donnée sur les espèce sédimenticoles, qui seraient les plus exposées.

## RESUMEN Y CONCLUSIONES

## 1. Resumen

### *1.1 Identidad, propiedades físicas y químicas y métodos analíticos*

La carbendazima es una sustancia sólida cristalina de color blanco y acción fungicida sistémica que pertenece a la familia del bencimidazol. Su punto de fusión es de unos 250 °C y tiene una presión de vapor de < 1 x $10^{-7}$ Pa (< 1 x $10^{-9}$ mbar). Es prácticamente insoluble en agua (8 mg/litro) a pH 7 y 20 °C. Es un compuesto estable en condiciones de almacenamiento normales.

Los análisis de las muestras de residuos y del medio ambiente se realizan mediante extracción con un disolvente orgánico y purificación del extracto obtenido utilizando un procedimiento de reparto líquido-líquido. La valoración de los residuos se puede realizar mediante cromatografía líquida de alto rendimiento o inmunoensayo.

### *1.2 Fuentes de exposición humana y ambiental*

La carbendazima es la sustancia más ampliamente utilizada de la familia de los fungicidas bencimidazólicos. Está formulada como dispersión acuosa, suspensión acuosa, gránulos fluidos dispersables en agua y polvo humectable.

### *1.3 Transporte, distribución y transformación en el medio ambiente*

En el medio ambiente, el benomilo se transforma rápidamente en carbendazima, con una semivida de 2 y 19 h en el agua y en el suelo, respectivamente. Por consiguiente, para la evaluación de los efectos sobre el medio ambiente son importantes los datos obtenidos de los estudios realizados con ambos compuestos.

La carbendazima se descompone en el medio ambiente, con una semivida de 6 a 12 meses en el suelo desnudo, de 3 a 6 meses en el césped y de 2 y 25 meses en el agua en condiciones aerobias y anaerobias, respectivamente. La descomposición se debe sobre todo a la acción de los microorganismos; el principal producto de su degradación es el 2-aminobencimidazol (2-AB), que luego se descompone de nuevo, también por la actividad microbiana. En la descomposición del benomilo marcado con un grupo fenilo con $^{14}C$, sólo el 9% del $^{14}C$ formó $CO_2$ durante un año de incubación, mientras que el resto del $^{14}C$ se recuperó sobre todo como carbendazima y en productos unidos a residuos. El destino de un posible producto de degradación (1,2-diaminobenceno) puede aclarar ulteriormente la vía de degradación de los fungicidas bencimidazólicos en el medio ambiente.

En estudios de campo y de columna se ha puesto de manifiesto que la carbendazima queda retenida en la capa superficial del suelo. Aunque no se dispone de datos sobre su adsorción en el suelo, es probable que ésta sea tan intensa como la del benomilo (los valores de $K_{oc}$ oscilan entre 1000 y 3600). Los valores del log $K_{ow}$ para el benomilo y la carbendazima son respectivamente 1,36 y 1,49.

En la evaluación realizada en un modelo de selección, basado en datos de adsorción y persistencia, se puso de manifiesto que no había riesgo de lixiviación. En los Estados Unidos se han efectuado análisis de agua de pozos que confirman esto, puesto que no se encontraron trazas de carbendazima en ninguno de los 212 pozos muestreados (no se dispone del límite de detección). Es de suponer que la escorrentía superficial del benomilo y la carbendazima se deba solamente al fungicida adsorbido en las partículas del suelo y que en el medio acuoso estén fuertemente adsorbidos en los sedimentos.

La carbendazima se hidroliza a 2-AB. Este es también el metabolito primario en el suelo y las plantas.

En los sistemas animales se metaboliza a (5-hidroxi-1H-bencimidazol-2-il)-carbamato (5-HBC) y otros metabolitos polares, que se excretan rápidamente. No se ha observado que la carbendazima se acumule en ningún sistema biológico.

### 1.4 Niveles medioambientales y exposición humana

No parece que se disponga de datos de vigilancia ambiental para la carbendazima. Sin embargo, los estudios realizados sobre su destino en el medio ambiente pueden resumirse como sigue.

Puesto que el benomilo y la carbendazima se mantienen estables en las plantas durante varias semanas, pueden pasar a los organismos que se alimentan de las hojas caídas. El suelo y los sedimentos pueden conservar residuos de carbendazima hasta tres años. Sin embargo, la fuerte adsorción de este compuesto en las partículas del suelo y en los sedimentos reduce la exposición de los organismos terrestres y acuáticos.

La principal fuente de exposición para la población humana general se debe a los residuos de benomilo y carbendazima en los cultivos alimentarios. En análisis de la exposición a través de los alimentos realizados en los Estados Unidos (benomilo y carbendazima combinados) y en los Países Bajos (con carbendazima) se obtuvo una ingesta media prevista de alrededor del 10 por ciento de la ingesta diaria admisible (IDA) recomendada, de 0,02 mg/kg de peso corporal para el benomilo y de 0,01 mg/kg de peso corporal para la carbendazima.

La exposición profesional durante el proceso de fabricación es inferior al valor umbral límite. Se considera que los trabajadores agrícolas que se ocupan de mezclar y cargar los plaguicidas o que entran en campos tratados con benomilo sufren exposición cutánea a unos mg de benomilo por hora. Esta forma de exposición se podría reducir con algún tipo de protección. Por otra parte, puesto que la absorción cutánea que cabe prever es baja, la probabilidad de que el benomilo tenga efectos tóxicos sistémicos a través de esta vía es muy escasa.

### 1.5 Cinética y metabolismo

La carbendazima se absorbe bien tras la exposición oral (80-85%), pero mucho menos después de una exposición cutánea. Una vez absorbida, se metaboliza formando numerosos compuestos en el organismo. Los principales metabolitos son el 5-HBC y los óxidos de 5,6-HOBC-N; otros menos son importantes el 5,6-DHBC-S y el 5,6-DHBC-G.

La distribución de la carbendazima en los tejidos demuestra la ausencia de bioconcentración. En la rata, la concentración más elevada tras su administración oral (< 1% de la dosis) se produjo en el hígado. Apareció carbendazima en las mitocondrias, el metabolito 5-HBC en el citosol y el 2-AB en los microsomas. Aunque se encontraron también carbendazima y sus metabolitos en el riñón de gallinas y de vacas, no se detectaron niveles significativos en otros tejidos. Tras suministrar carbendazima con el pienso a vacas lactantes, se encontraron pequeñas cantidades de 5-HBC y 4-HBC en la leche.

La carbendazima se excreta en la orina y las heces en un plazo de 72 h tras la dosificación oral en ratas.

En ratas y ratones, la administración de dosis altas de carbendazima en la dieta o con sonda afectó a ciertas enzimas de los microsomas. Se produjo inducción de la estireno-7,8-hidrolasa y de la epóxido-hidrolasa, mientras que se redujo la actividad de la hidroxicumarín-O-deetilasa. También se indujo la actividad de la glutatión-S-transferasa citosólica.

## 1.6 Efectos en los mamíferos de laboratorio y en sistemas de prueba in vitro

### 1.6.1 Exposición única

La carbendazima tiene una toxicidad aguda baja. Los valores de la $DL_{50}$ oscilan entre > 2000 y 15 000 mg/kg en una amplia variedad de animales de experimentación y de vías de administración. Sin embargo, se han observado efectos reproductivos adversos significativos en la salud tras una exposición única (véase la sección 1.6.5).

### 1.6.2 Exposición de corta duración

La administración de carbendazima en la dieta durante un período de hasta 90 días produjo efectos leves en el peso del hígado de las ratas hembras expuestas a 360 mg/kg de peso corporal al día. En un estudio de alimentación con sonda a ratas durante 90 días, el NOEL fue de 16 mg/kg por día, basado en la hepatotoxicidad. Los estudios de alimentación de corta duración en perros no se consideraron adecuados para establecer un NOEL. En un estudio cutáneo de 10 días en conejos no se detectó toxicidad sistémica con la única dosis ensayada (200 mg/kg).

### 1.6.3 Irritación y sensibilización cutánea y ocular

La aplicación a la piel de conejos y cobayos no produjo irritación o sensibilización cutánea. Tras la aplicación a los ojos de conejos se observó una irritación conjuntival moderada o ligera.

### 1.6.4 Exposición prolongada

En ratas macho y hembra a las que se administraron 2500 mg/kg de alimentos se registró una disminución del número de eritrocitos y de los valores de la hemoglobina y el hematocrito. No se observó ninguna toxicidad de tipo hepático. Las ratas macho a las que se administraron 2500 mg/kg de alimentos o más presentaron un aumento marginal de la atrofia testicular y la prostatitis. El NOEL en las ratas es de 500 mg/kg de alimentos. En perros que recibieron una dieta con 500 mg de carbendazima por kg de alimentos durante un año o más se observó aumento del colesterol sérico, elevación de la actividad de la fosfatasa alcalina y otras indicaciones de hepatotoxicidad. El NOEL en perros es de 300 mg/kg de alimentos.

### 1.6.5 Reproducción, embriotoxicidad y teratogenicidad

La carbendazima no tuvo ningún efecto adverso en la reproducción cuando se administró a ratas en un estudio de reproducción de tres generaciones a dosis de hasta 500 mg/kg de alimentos. Se registró una reducción de la fecundidad masculina en las ratas a las que se administró carbendazima (200 mg/kg por día) con sonda durante 85 días. Con una dosis de 50 mg/kg de peso corporal al día en este estudio disminuyó considerablemente el número de espermatozoides en el epidídimo.

Tras la administración a ratas de una dosis oral única de 100 mg/kg de peso corporal, el examen histológico puso de manifiesto una interrupción temprana (0-2 días) de la espermatogénesis, con oclusión de los conductos eferentes y un aumento del peso de los testículos. En este estudio de dosis única no se observó ningún efecto con 50 mg/kg. Los efectos se mantuvieron hasta transcurridos 70 días en ratas tratadas con 400 mg/kg.

La carbendazima provocó un aumento de las malformaciones y las anomalías en las ratas administrada a dosis diarias superiores a 10 mg/kg en los días 7-16 de la gestación. En conejas se produjo un ligero descenso de la tasa de implantación en dosis de 20 y 125 mg/kg por día administradas en los días 7-19 de la gestación, y un aumento de la incidencia de la reabsorción a 125 mg/kg por día. Se observó toxicidad materna con dosis de 20 y de 125 mg/kg por día en ratas y conejos, respectivamente.

Además del descenso de la tasa de gestaciones y del aumento de las reabsorciones precoces en la rata, se produjo una reducción significativa del peso del feto con dosis de 20 y 90 mg/kg por día, y un incremento significativo de las malformaciones fetales con la dosis de 90 mg/kg por día. Estas consistieron fundamentalmente en hidrocefalia, microftalmia, anoftalmia, malformaciones escapulares y del esqueleto axial (fusiones vertebrales, costales y esternebrales, exencefalia, hemivértebras e hiperplasia costal). Sin embargo, en los conejos no aparecieron malformaciones significativas.

### 1.6.6 Mutagenicidad y otros efectos finales afines

Los ensayos realizados en sistemas de mamíferos y no mamíferos *in vitro* e *in vivo* y en células somáticas, así como en células germinales, demuestran que la carbendazima no tiene interacción con el ADN celular, no induce mutaciones puntuales y tampoco produce mutaciones de las células germinales.

Sin embargo, la carbendazima provoca aberraciones cromosómicas numéricas (aneuploidía o poliploidía) en sistemas experimentales *in vitro* e *in vivo*.

### 1.6.7 Carcinogenicidad

La administración de benomilo y carbendazima con los alimentos a ratones CD-1 y suizos SPF dio lugar a un aumento de la incidencia de tumores hepatocelulares.

Un estudio de carcinogenicidad de la carbendazima con ratones CD-1 puso de manifiesto un aumento estadísticamente significativo, relacionado con la dosis, de la neoplasia hepatocelular en las hembras. También se observó un aumento estadísticamente significativo en los machos tratados con una dosis de nivel medio (1500 mg/kg de alimentos), pero no en los que recibieron dosis altas, a causa de la elevada mortalidad. Un estudio sobre la carcinogenicidad de la carbendazima en una raza de ratones genéticamente relacionada con la anterior, los ratones SPF (raza aleatoria suiza), con dosis de 0, 150, 300 y 1000 mg/kg de alimentos (que se aumentó a 5000 mg/kg durante el estudio), mostró un aumento de la incidencia de adenomas y carcinomas hepatocelulares combinados. Un tercer estudio realizado en ratones NMRKf con dosis de 0, 50, 150, 300 y 1000 mg de carbendazima por kg de alimentos (que se aumentó a 5000 mg/kg durante el estudio) no puso de manifiesto efectos carcinogénicos. El benomilo y la carbendazima provocaron tumores hepáticos en dos razas de ratones (CD-1 y SPF), ambas con un elevado índice de tumores hepáticos espontáneos. En cambio, la carbendazima no es carcinogénica en ratones NMRKf, que tienen un índice bajo de este tipo de tumores espontáneos.

Los estudios de carcinogenicidad del benomilo y la carbendazima en ratas fueron negativos.

### .6.8 Mecanismo de toxicidad, modo de acción

Los efectos biológicos del benomilo y la carbendazima se deben a su interacción con los microtúbulos celulares. Estas estructuras intervienen en funciones esenciales, como la división celular, que inhiben el benomilo y la carbendazima. La toxicidad de estos productos en los mamíferos está vinculada a una disfunción microtubular.

El benomilo y la carbendazima, al igual que otros compuestos del bencimidazol, tienen una toxicidad selectiva para distintas especies, que se explica, por lo menos en parte, porque el benomilo y la carbendazima se unen de manera distinta a los microtúbulos de las especies específicas en las que actúan y en las que no.

### 1.7 Efectos en el ser humano

No se ha informado de efectos adversos para la salud humana.

### 1.8 Efectos en otros organismos en el laboratorio y en el medio ambiente

Con las dosis de aplicación recomendadas, la carbendazima tiene pocos efectos sobre la actividad microbiana del suelo. Se han notificado algunos efectos adversos sobre ciertos tipos de hongos.

La $CE_{50}$ a las 72 horas para el alga verde *Selenastrum capricornutum*, basada en el crecimiento total, se calculó en 1,3 mg/litro; la NOEC fue de 0,5 mg/litro. La toxicidad de la carbendazima para los invertebrados acuáticos y los peces varía ampliamente, con una $CL_{50}$ a las 96 h que oscila entre 0,007 mg/litro para *Ictalurus punctatus* y 5,5 mg/litro para *Lepomis macrochirus*. En una prueba de 21 días con *Daphnia magna*, el comienzo de la reproducción se retrasó considerablemente con 0,025 mg/litro; la NOEC fue de 0,013 mg/litro.

La carbendazima es tóxica para las lombrices de tierra en experimentos de laboratorio con una exposición a concentraciones normales y con las dosis de aplicación recomendadas en el campo. Es "relativamente no tóxica" para las abejas de miel y su toxicidad es baja para las aves.

## 2. Conclusiones

El benomilo causa sensibilización cutánea en el ser humano. Tanto el benomilo como la carbendazima representan un riesgo muy pequeño de intoxicación aguda. Dados los niveles de exposición actuales y el bajo índice de absorción cutánea de estos dos compuestos, no es probable que puedan tener efectos de toxicidad sistémica en la población general o en personas expuestas profesionalmente. Estas son las conclusiones que se pueden sacar de los datos obtenidos en animales y de los limitados datos sobre el ser humano de que se dispone, pero estas extrapolaciones están respaldadas por el conocimiento del modo de acción de la carbendazima y el benomilo en especies en las que actúan y en las que no.

Una mayor clarificación del mecanismo de toxicidad de ambos compuestos en los mamíferos permitirá quizás definir mejor los niveles sin efectos observados. El estudio de su unión a los microtúbulos de las células destinatarias (tejidos testicular y embrionario) facilitará la comparación entre distintas especies.

La carbendazima se adsorbe fuertemente en la materia orgánica del suelo, que la conserva durante un período de hasta tres años. Persiste en la superficie de las hojas y, por consiguiente, en las hojas caídas. Se ha demostrado que las dosis recomendadas de aplicación afectan negativamente a las lombrices de tierra (con efectos sobre la población y la reproducción). No se dispone de datos acerca de sus efectos sobre otros artrópodos del suelo o de la maleza, que estarían igualmente expuestos.

No es probable que se pueda observar en el medio ambiente la elevada toxicidad demostrada en las pruebas de laboratorio para los organismos acuáticos, debido a la baja biodisponibilidad de los residuos de carbendazima unidos a los sedimentos. Sin embargo, no se dispone de información acerca de sus efectos en las especies que viven en los sedimentos, que sufrirían la exposición más intensa.